Let's Try Real Food

Let's Try Real Food

A Practical Guide to Nutrition and Good Health

by Ethel Hulbert Renwick

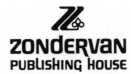

ZONDERVAN
PUBLISHING HOUSE

OF THE ZONDERVAN CORPORATION | GRAND RAPIDS, MICHIGAN 49506

Unless otherwise indicated, Scripture references in New Testament are from *The New International Version* New Testament. © 1973 by New York Bible Society International. Used by permission. The Old Testament references are from *Revised Standard Version*.

LET'S TRY REAL FOOD
© 1976 by The Zondervan Corporation
Grand Rapids, Michigan

Sixth printing 1982

ISBN 0-310-31861-0

Library of Congress Cataloging in Publication Data

Renwick, Ethel Hulbert.
    Let's try real food.
    1. Nutrition.   2. Diet.   3. Stewardship, Christian.
I. Title.
TX357.R46   613.2   76-11850

Printed in the United States of America

In memory of
ALICIA VEREIDE DAVISON
who was not only a constant source
of inspiration to me, as she was to
countless others, but an encouragement
in my undertaking this book.

Contents

Part 6—Could This Be You?

Part 7—Nutrition as Christian Stewardship

Acknowledgments

I wish to express my deep gratitude to my husband; our two sons, George and Bob; our daughter, Margo; and our good friend Carol Sippy, for their supportive interest, their invaluable interaction, and their part in the formation of this book.

Introduction

May the God of peace himself sanctify you wholly; and
may your spirit and soul and body be kept sound and
blameless at the coming of the Lord Jesus Christ.
1 Thessalonians 5:23, RSV

Several years of my life were spent traveling leisurely
throughout the world with my family. It was our good fortune
to have traveled before the spread of communism, before the
rush of industrialization to many of the more remote areas of
the world, and before the phenomenal escalation of tourism
which came with the acceleration of air travel. All I witnessed—
on freighters through tropical isles, on elephant-back through
jungle terrain, on narrow railways across distant landscapes,
and on all manner of motor vehicles through primitive as well
as highly civilized areas of the world—brought into focus for
me the basic necessities of life and health.

As I observed, studied, and compared the peoples of the
world, and as I became vividly aware of the fundamental necessities for physical well-being, I came to realize how tragically
ignorant we Americans are of these necessities.

Because of our influence overseas, Americans have a
special responsibility to be aware and informed. Christians in
America bear even greater responsibilities because of our concern for growth, wholeness, and effective functioning. Yet we
have failed to live up to these responsibilities. Our ignorance
of how to build and maintain healthy bodies, together with our
consequent failure to take action for the betterment of ourselves
and others, is a serious indictment against us. We are hearing
more and more about the "whole" person, but Christians ignore the area of physical vitality.

Dr. Paul Tournier, the eminent Swiss physician who has
contributed substantially to the layman's understanding of psychiatry in the Christian context, states that "Many illnesses
occur neither abruptly nor by chance, but rather have been
prepared through years of a comportment contrary to the laws
of life." [1] Using Tournier's phraseology, I would suggest that
many illnesses and physical weaknesses in America today have

been prepared, through the last one hundred years, by eating habits and an accelerated pace of living which are contrary to the laws of life.

We are paying heavily for this departure from what God intended for His creation. Some of us may have average health, but how many of us have exuberant health? How many of us have more minor illnesses and less stamina than we should? To what extent do we drive ourselves on what we wrongly call "nervous energy" and rationalize the overextension of our personal resources as being necessary? Our less than excellent health reduces our patience, efficiency, emotional stability, and effectiveness as God's people. Consequently, many of us break down in one way or another.

What are we saying to others, especially to young people, about our responsibility for our personal, physical resources and about the possibilities for strength and complete wholeness? As long as we fail to appreciate and nourish ourselves physically, what kind of examples are we?

I think we are apt to take all scriptural references to the body as if they concern only its moral abuse. For example: "May the God of peace himself sanctify you wholly; and may your spirit and soul and body be kept sound and blameless at the coming of the Lord Jesus Christ" (1 Thess. 5:23, RSV). Note that the words used here are *sound* and *blameless. Blameless* would refer to the absence of immoral acts, whereas *sound* would mean health and strength. A sound body is as capable of being immoral as a weak body, so it would seem that Scripture is saying Christians are expected to take care of their bodies from a health standpoint as an act of stewardship. Just as spiritual soundness and growth are essential, so are physical soundness and growth, and both influence emotional and mental health.

Nutrition is essential to physical soundness and growth. I believe that most of us have, perhaps unwittingly, for too long ignored nutrition. This neglect has been to our personal detriment, our nation's detriment, and, therefore, to the detriment of God's plan for us. The Christian community contributes to this ignorance by not accepting and advocating an alternative style of eating and living. We are shirking vital responsibilities.

This book deals with these responsibilities. I address it with loving concern to the Christian community. Many of us purchase, cook, and plan food for our families; some of us sell food or run organizations that serve food; a few of us prescribe food; and all of us eat food. Consequently, none of us escapes the responsibility of properly nourishing the body God has given us. We must ask ourselves two important questions: What does what we eat have to do with being a Christian? And, are we eating real food?

PART 1

Our Neglected Responsibility

Do you not know that your body is a temple of the Holy Spirit, who is in you, whom you have received from God? You are not your own; you were bought at a price. Therefore honor God with your body.

1 Corinthians 6:19, 20

Chapter 1

The Care of the Body

I was made aware of good nutrition when I was very young. My mother, who was born in the United States but was brought up in Europe, had always been interested in and studied food. She herself did not cook, but she could tell you in four languages what was wrong with almost any dish. With her knowledge of the good foods of many countries, our daily meals were interesting as well as carefully cooked. Early in life I learned to abhor overly cooked vegetables, pasty soups, poorly made sauces, overly sweetened foods, and soft drinks. The only desserts we had were fresh fruits, homemade gelatins and puddings, imported cheeses, and homemade ice creams made with certified raw milk.

When I was still young, my father became severely ill, and the top medical men in Chicago gave him from six months to a year to live. My father decided that if the medical profession could offer nothing further, he would turn to nutrition. He studied it avidly and taught our entire family (and the cook, of course) his discoveries about good nutrition. I will never forget the pancakes we had which were made of seven whole-grain flours—they were superb! I soon learned that gourmet cooking could encompass the best natural foods in the world.

However, the important point is that my father lived for many years. He was able to enjoy his fishing boat in Florida every winter, and he had trained his cook on the boat to prepare the same wholesome food which had become his complete new regimen. In our family we saw living proof of what eating God's natural provisions could do for us, even when the medical profession declared someone beyond help.

With this background, then, it is no wonder that during our numerous travels I was keenly interested in the eating habits, life styles, and consequent health of the various peoples of this earth. It also follows that I became even more aware of our own national diet and health in the United States. Over the years I have watched with alarm as our country's diet has become increasingly worse; and yet the majority of people are unaware of this. Then I started looking at the problem from a Christian perspective, and I realized that we as Christians are contributing to our national dilemma, thereby ignoring an important dimension of stewardship—the proper care of the bodies God gave us. This reponsibility we can do something about right here and now.

Genesis 1 states, "And God saw everything that he had made, and behold, it was very good" (v. 31). What is creation today? Polluted. Objects of pollution are air, water, soil, sound, and food. And to this we may certainly add man's mind and soul. The fruit of those trying to get along without God and live by a code devised by man for his convenience—but not for his ultimate health and happiness—abounds in every area of society. This fruit comes in the form of abuses in drugs, alcohol, sex, and food. And these in turn put an enormous burden on society: broken people, broken homes, deserted or runaway children, emotional problems, crime, and ill health—an alarming situation.

This book will deal at some length with food pollution and food abuse and will touch on consequences of our hectic, overcrowded lives. Our acceptance of this life style has led us to neglect our bodies and abuse God's natural order, and it has contributed to many of our current problems. We abuse our bodies through overwork and by the manner in which we deal with the pressures of life. We do not distinguish between productive work and overwork which results in overextending our-

selves. We abuse our bodies through poor diet. Christians neglect good nutrition and ignore physical truths. We ask for
health, but we neglect to learn about the nutrients for health.
We do not recognize the adulteration of food for the sake of
profit by the manufacturer, and we do not distinguish between
fad and the natural order. There is much we can do to correct
the situation, and it is our responsibility to do so.

The Pace of Life

One of the great ills of our society is that Americans make
outrageous demands upon their bodies by overwork. The work
ethic, being at the very core of America, is taken to an extreme
and rationalized as worthy, even noble. America has forgotten
how to relax. No wonder youth rebels at this. Can we not say
that the same attitude toward work drives the Christian—the
layman in business, the Christian worker in his endeavor—
beyond the physical limits with which he is endowed?

Many times I have been asked why Christians have breakdowns. I know there can be several reasons, but it seems clear
that many Christians break down from a misguided attitude
toward work and too little observance of rest. Many of us do
not know how to stop long enough to enjoy and appreciate both
the beauty of life around us and the stillness of contemplation.

In America today there is little respect for the privacy of
others which, in itself, robs us of regular opportunities to relax,
to meditate, to reassess, and to accomplish the personal necessities of life at leisure. As a friend of mine says, "Come apart
before you fall apart." I believe that many of us will fall apart
if we do not operate according to the physical limitations God
has given us or eat the things He has provided to keep our
bodies strong enough to cope with the pressures in which we
find ourselves.

Pressure is not a recent phenomenon, and we should be
able to respond to quite a lot of it, constructive or harmful,
without adverse effects. Our Lord lived under tremendous emotional and mental pressure: He lived knowing He was a threat
to those in power, and He knew that what lay ahead of Him
was crucifixion at the hands of those He had come to save. He
had to contend with daily pressures of many kinds: the greed
of men, crooked business, corrupt politics, licentiousness,

crime, debauchery, drunkenness, sexual perversion, godless-
ness, and He had to attack the religionists and the establishment. He lived within all these pressures to call people out of
their legalisms and empty, graft-filled temples, out of their
blind and corrupt societal practices, into a life of forgiveness,
redemption, love, freedom, purpose, fulfillment, and peace. In
the life of Jesus we see many examples of what we today call
pressure, indicating that we must not fear pressures but must
be prepared to face them with a clear perspective and a strong
constitution.

What I see in myself and so many others is that we work
hard to have a good attitude and we count heavily on God's
grace, but we are worn out. We take on a great deal more than
we can do, which means, of course, we are not doing everything as well as we should. I have seen many Christians live
as though God depended on them alone and had no other way
of getting things done. God does not expect man to do all the
work he sees around him, and one of our earliest directives to
this effect comes from Jethro, Moses' father-in-law, who remon-
strated with Moses for trying by himself to tell everyone the
statutes of God. Jethro said, "What you are doing is not good.
You and the people with you will wear yourselves out, for this
thing is too heavy for you; you are not able to perform it alone"
(Exod. 18:17, 18). This verse belongs in large letters in many
homes and offices.

Obviously we are not supposed to undertake more than
we can do well while maintaining our health. The first ones to
suffer from our overtaxing ourselves are the ones who should
have our first concern—our families. If we see no one to do
whatever job we think needs to be taken care of, we can trust
the Lord: His ways are higher than our ways. We seek the will
of God, yet it is hard to believe that ignoring our physical limits
and being too worn out to function well—even becoming ill—is
in His will for us. It is difficult to keep a perspective on a
situation we are caught up in, but it would seem to me that no
matter how important something looks, or how gratifying, it is
of no account if it is not God's will for us. We harm ourselves
and, as Jethro so wisely said, other people.

When we have overextended ourselves, we are not sharp
mentally, we often set our nerves on edge without realizing it,

we have less patience, poor judgment, and our emotional reactions become less controllable. When we overdo, we are not running on "nervous energy," as the expression goes, but we are burning up our body chemistry. It is not God's plan for us to live like this. We all know from experience that God sees us through emergencies most miraculously; He gives us extra strength, keenness of mind, and stability. But it is certainly not His plan for us to live on a regular basis the way we do when we are called on to act in an emergency. I think we delude ourselves into thinking we are necessary to a situation beyond the limitations of our health. It is here that the Christian community can teach—not just mention—pacing ourselves, praying, and meditating.

Alvin Toffler, in his astounding book *Future Shock,* gives a mind-boggling description of the wound-up, hurried man of today and makes the following poignant observation:

> The pace of life is frequently commented upon by ordinary people. Yet, oddly enough, it has received almost no attention from either psychologists or sociologists. This is a gaping inadequacy in the behavioral sciences, for the pace of life profoundly influences behavior, provoking strong and contrasting reactions from different people. It is, in fact, not too much to say that the pace of life draws a line through humanity, dividing us into camps, triggering bitter misunderstanding between parent and child, between Madison Avenue and Main Street, between men and women, between American and European, between East and West.[1]

The pace of life has been commented on by several deeply spiritual Christians, but the rest of us in the Christian community seem to have overlooked the example of the unhurried life of Jesus. Is it any wonder that some youths, seeking a better way of life, look elsewhere?

How We Eat

Overtaxing ourselves by rushing around and spreading ourselves too thin leads us into another evil. People who are this busy are usually eating neither regularly nor well. Most of us have to discipline ourselves to take time to eat properly. This adds to fatigue and tears down the nervous system. Our general well-being has an enormous influence on our dispositions and our approach to problems. It can affect every relationship. It is time we learned, lived, and taught more about God's natural order and His natural provisions for us if we want to be as whole, as fit, and as useful as possible.

Inasmuch as the Bible uses physical truths to explain spiritual truths, I think we can assume that the physical truths to which the Bible refers are valid. Spiritual truths cannot be ignored without cost to the one who chooses to ignore them. Likewise, physical truths cannot be ignored without cost to the one who chooses to ignore them. Under physical truths are the laws of good nutrition. To go against these laws is detrimental, yet, for some unknown reason, the majority of Christians feel perfectly justified in doing so.

Besides giving heed to God's natural laws, the Christian community must listen to what nutritionists are saying. There are at least fifty years of responsible, documented research to rely on in the field of nutrition. One source of information is the International College of Applied Nutrition, which has been accumulating valuable research in the way of scientific articles for a half century. Their journal is the voice of a growing nucleus of physicians, dentists, veterinarians, agronomists, bio-chemists, and nutritionists. The publications of the International Academy of Preventive Medicine are another source, and there are many books on the subject which have been written by competent men and women in the field and are available at most bookstores.

There is no excuse for ignorance. However, just as many people try to get along in their adult life on a few childhood recollections and impressions of Christianity, so many try to get along in life with a stunted knowledge of food. Most of us have only a vague idea of today's food produce, our body requirements, and proper nutrition. God's provisions for physical nourishment, for which we are to give thanks daily, are not taught within the Christian context.

The shelves of the leading bookstores are lined with the teachings on diets of various religions and cults, and they are attracting a surprising number of our youth, as well as some older Americans. We should not wonder at this. The Christian community has offered nothing. Nowhere have I found a book on the Christian's responsibility—his sense of stewardship—in regard to his diet. How many Christians are conscious of whether they are partaking of God's provisions or man's adulterated and impoverished substitute? Very few.

Why are there so few Christians who are aware of what they are eating? Whenever I mention good nutrition to anyone, men or women, they usually want to set me straight about how well they eat and how particular they are about what they feed their families. I know they are sincere; they really believe they are doing a conscientious job. However, as many of them elaborate on their diets, I can see they have a superficial knowledge of nutrition. Then there are many Christians who are, or have been, in some aspect of the food business; I number among them. They run honest, efficient, successful restaurants, groceries, or distributorships, and they meet the demand of their customers as best they can. However, meeting the demands of customers and being successful are not the Christian's only concerns and certainly not his criteria. We are to be concerned with whether we are contributing to people's well-being.

How is it then that we are not supplying the best possible nourishment God has provided to keep us well and strong? The answers to this are manifold, and I go into them in some detail in succeeding chapters. However, to sum them up generally, I would point out that "in the beginning" (Gen. 1:1), and for most generations to follow, God's creatures ate the food He provided for them. It was not necessary for them to have any knowledge about food at all. Today, however, each of us has to be knowledgeable because man has altered these provisions.

What We Eat

Few of us live off the land, so we are subject to what the producer does to our food. We are also misled by what he says about what he produces and wishes to sell to us. Furthermore, we not only turn for advice to medical men who do not study nutrition, but we are influenced by those among them who express derogatory and uneducated opinions of learned biochemists and nutritionists. Lastly, our government sanctions the alterations in food from the field and feed lot, through all the processing, to the marketplace, and to our tables.

Professor Ross Hume Hall of McMaster University Health

Sciences Centre at Hamilton, Ontario, is a man of extensive experience in both cancer research and the biology of growth and development. He has also worked in the field of nutrition and has made a profound and penetrating study of the processes which have been set in motion by the mechanical world to subjugate the organic world. By the term *organic world* he means all natural processes. He has written an analytical and scholarly book, *Food for Nought: The Decline in Nutrition,* which grew out of this study. It points out that the organic world is being subjugated because no comprehensive, in-depth assessment of the startling transformation we have gone through has been made by those to whom the public looks and trusts to protect them. Dr. Hall puts into focus for us the tyranny of unmonitored technology of which we are allowing ourselves to become victims.

> Nourishment of the American populace has undergone a startling transformation since World War II. A highly individual system of growing and marketing food has been transformed into a gigantic, highly integrated service system in which the object is not to nourish or even feed, but to force an ever-increasing consumption of fabricated products.... Man can never be more than what he eats, and one would expect that a phenomenon with such profound effects on health and well-being as a radically changed system of supplying nourishment would be thoroughly documented and assessed by the scientific community. Such is not the case. The transformation has gone unmarked by government agencies and learned bodies. Government agencies, recipients of the public trust charged with protecting and improving the public's food, operate as if the technology of food fabrication rested in pre-World War II days. Scientific bodies, supported by public funds and charged with assessing and improving the public's health, ignore completely the results of contemporary methods of producing and marketing food.[2]

Have we not been misled far beyond anything we had imagined? In any event, few Christians are aware of what they are eating, serving, and selling. But we need not continue in ignorance or partial ignorance.

God provided correct nourishment for the growth and health of the body. Therefore, to pray for a healthy body and refuse to study nutrition and the effect technology has on it today is as illogical as praying for spiritual growth and refusing to read the Bible and other inspiring, instructive books on the Christian life. We dare not continue to ignore God's physical rules for our health and growth any more than we dare disregard His spiritual laws.

A great deal of ill health is due to what we eat. Do we pray for health and healing and eat poorly?

Chapter 2

The Civilized Diet—Before and After

Dr. George M. Briggs, professor of nutrition at the University of California, says candidly, "The typical American diet is a national disaster." He contends that the average American maintains a terrible diet and that if he fed it to pigs or cows, without adding vitamins and other supplements, he could wipe out the livestock industry. Dr. Briggs claims that there is much malnutrition in this country among rich and poor alike and that it shows up in many different ways—hunger, nutrient deficiencies, high incidence of anemia, increased infections, underweight and overweight, severe dental problems, reduced growth, needless problems in pregnancy and with infants, shortened life spans, and even behavioral and mental problems in children and adults. He is of the opinion that diabetes, heart disease, alcoholism, and other great problems are related in part to poor nutrition. It is no surprise that Dr. Briggs believes that adequate nutritious food is not only essential to good health—it is a matter of life and death.

Nutritionists have been telling us this for the forty years I have been reading their books and listening to their lectures. It is now being expressed more widely, but still from too few. Many competent nutritionists are convinced, as is Dr. Briggs,

13

that the basic reasons for our dilemma are that our national leaders do not recognize the need for nutrition and that too few people with proper nutrition training hold key positions in our schools and food industries (I would add to this, our clinics and our churches). Dr. Briggs does, however, place most of the responsibility on the individual when he says that the fault lies largely in ourselves for the kind of foods we eat and demand on the shelves of our grocery stores.

I consider this an indictment against the Christian *community*—not only our pastors and ruling bodies, but the entire body of believers. Christians do suffer from breakdowns, disorders, and diseases, and though we can excuse ourselves by saying we did not know the role nutrition plays in all these problems, we must admit that we consider our bodies to be the temple of the Holy Spirit and that we neither investigated good nutrition nor took a stand on it. We need nutritionists in key positions in our churches and Christian organizations, especially when most of our nation's leaders and educators are shirking their responsibility in this vital field.

God's Provisions

To more clearly comprehend that our national diet is a departure from what God intended, we have only to look at our diet before and after it was "civilized," as depicted by Dr. Weston A. Price in his book *Nutrition and Physical Degeneration,* which was first published in 1939 and again in 1970. This book should have shaken our nation and radically changed its eating habits. The *Journal of the American Dental Association* claimed that the book was "one of the outstanding books in dental literature in recent years." The *Pittsburgh Courier* said of the book:

> Dr. Price, a Cleveland dentist, circled the globe studying the relation of nutrition to health and degeneration. He found that whenever our "tin can" civilization had touched the natives they had terrible teeth and all of our loathsome degenerative diseases. He is honest enough to admit the superior culture of these "uncivilized" people, and he contends that unless we adopt their wisdom we will perish.

Earnest Albert Hooton, professor of anthropology at Harvard University, says in his foreword to the book:

Since we have known for a long time that savages have excellent teeth and that civilized men have terrible teeth, it seems to me that we have been extraordinarily stupid in concentrating all of our attention upon the task of finding out why our teeth are so poor, without ever bothering to learn why savage teeth are good. Dr. Weston Price seems to be the only person who possesses the scientific horse sense to supplement his knowledge of the probable causes of dental disease with a study of the dietary regimens which are associated with dental health. . . . [he] has found out why primitive men have good teeth and why their teeth go bad when they become "civilized." But he has not stopped there: he has gone on to apply his knowledge acquired from savages to the problems of their less intelligent civilized brothers. For I think that we must admit that if savages know enough to eat the things which keep their teeth healthy, they are more intelligent in dietary matters than we are. So, I consider that Dr. Price has written what is often called "a profoundly significant book." [1]

Had Dr. Price's book shaken the nation when it was first published, our children and grandchildren would have better teeth and better physical and mental health today. As made clear in Dr. Price's book, poor teeth and malformed dental arches are the first signs of physical degeneration and "our loathsome degenerative diseases," to quote the *Pittsburgh Courier's* apt description of what ensues. Our nation and the civilized world had all the evidence they needed in the detailed findings carefully reported and photographed by Dr. Price, as well as by Sir Robert McCarrison[2] in India, in regard to the health of peoples of this world before the white man's diet of sugar, refined flour, and canned goods was introduced to them.

The uninformed are apt to say that it was not the change the natives made in their diet which caused the degeneration in their health, but the change they made in their living habits when civilization crept in. However, the natives who started adding sugar and refined flour to their diets *lived exactly as they always had.* Not all natives came to the ports and worked for the white man there, but the food introduced by the white man went back to the villages and was carried from tribe to tribe, often for trading purposes. Physical degeneration set in and was, as we ourselves witnessed, more and more pronounced as new generations were born.

The scientific findings of these doctors did, indeed, bear out what my family had observed of primitive people in various parts of the world, and, interestingly enough, we covered almost all the same areas. Our conclusion was that man, no matter where he lived or what his occupation, suffered severely when departing from what God had supplied in the way of food, and that the departure in every case was caused by the introduction of the white man's diet of refined flour and sugar. We saw clearly that our missionaries who went to all parts of the world to carry the gospel and to educate the illiterate needed more and more medical missionaries working alongside them because of what we "civilized" people were doing to undermine the health of the natives.

Wilmon Menard, anthropologist, sociologist, and writer, who spent many years of his life in the South Pacific, himself witnessed what he calls "civilization's kiss of death." He records a penetrating account of what took place among the Polynesians of the Marquesas Islands which verifies that the white man's adulterated diet is the cause of physical degeneration. Mr. Menard quotes Herman Melville's description of the Marquesans in 1841: "I was especially struck by the physical strength and beauty they displayed ... in beauty of form they surpassed anything I had seen ... free from blemish ... a sculptor's model." [3] Civilization came to the Marquesans, and they replaced their natural food with polished rice, tinned foods, and confections. Degeneration set in, and a population of about 100,000 dwindled to a sickly 2500. This was due, Mr. Menard says, to cash paid for their copra crops and the attendant prestige value the natives placed on imported European goods. Then came the day when the price of copra dropped, poverty set in, and the natives were forced back to their original simple but highly nutritious diet. The result: a return to health, few or no dental caries, and dazzling white teeth. The population started increasing instead of decreasing, and they were a healthy people again. On the coast where some of the people were still subjected to the white man's diet, the signs of degeneration continued.

Dr. Price made some interesting observations in Africa besides the usual findings of good health among the people before their exposure to modernized diets. In thirty primitive tribes north of Mombassa (in Kenya, Ethiopia, and so forth) with whom Dr. Price came in contact, he found the natives constitutionally immune to the diseases the white man contracts in this area: dysentery, malaria, typhoid fever, sleeping sickness, and others. Yet, when the natives of the primitive tribes adopted modern civilizations, they, too, became susceptible to those diseases and to tooth decay. Dr. Price also quotes a Dr. Anderson who was in charge of a government hospital in Kenya; Anderson assured Price that the primitive people of that district did not suffer from appendicitis, gall bladder trouble, cystitis, or duodenal ulcers, and that malignancy was rare.

Dr. Price gives many examples of diet among the different tribes in Africa, from the Negroid to the Arab and others who are characterized by their superb physical development and high intelligence. Throughout the centuries, their food has varied according to locale. Some tribes depend largely upon milk, meat, and blood (extracted from the jugular vein of the animal by a unique and antiseptic process), reinforced with vegetables and fruit. Others within reach of Lake Victoria or streams obtain large quantities of fish which constitute an important part of their diet, together with sweet potatoes and whole-grain cereals.

Several tribes neighboring Ethiopia are agriculturists, growing corn, beans, millet, sweet potatoes, bananas, Kafir corn, and other whole grains, which are their chief articles of food. What was particularly interesting to me was that the tribes living on vegetables alone were not as well built as the tribes using dairy products liberally or fish from the lakes and streams; they had been dominated because they possessed less courage and resourcefulness. My own observation has always been—in studying and in observing firsthand the various peoples of the world—that protein is valuable in the diet worldwide, and that strict vegetarians who eliminate dairy products as well as meat from their diet are less strong and less robust even under the most ideal conditions. Dr. Price's conclusions are similar to mine. He points out that Uganda, for instance, has been called the Garden of Eden because of its abundance of fresh water, fish, and animal life; natives of Uganda, besides being strong, are unusually intelligent.

One of the most efficiently organized mission schools in

Africa asked Dr. Price to help them solve a serious problem: why the families who had grown up in the mission and government schools were not as strong physically as those who had not had contact with them. The scourge, of course, was modern civilization.

Dr. Price found the same evidence among the Alaskan Eskimos and the Indians of Northern Canada where he could still find isolated tribes. The Forest Indians had superb health and lived among an abundance of wild animal life and vegetation. Wherever Indians were living on their native foods, chiefly moose and caribou meat, physical development—including facial dental arch—was superb, with nearly complete immunity to tooth decay. Wherever the Indians had access to the modern foods of commerce, Dr. Price said that the dental conditions were extremely bad. He found the same true of the Seminoles in the Everglades of Florida who were, in the thirties, still largely beyond contact with the white civilization and lived on native foods. They produced magnificent teeth and dental arches. Needless to say, today, the Seminoles, who have been living in contact with modern civilization and its food, suffer from rampant decay.

The State of Our Health

What is the result of the civilized diet of our nation? The result is that we are a sick nation. We must face this reality. Too many of us live under the illusion that we are not only the best-fed nation in the world, but the healthiest. The United World Health Organization made a survey in 1968 which revealed that the United States ranks twenty-fifth in male life expectancy and fourteenth in female life expectancy. Statistics are misleading. We are told we live longer, but the statistics only work that way because fewer babies die now under the age of five. In the book *Supernutrition* we learn that "contrary to popular belief, neither the maximum life span nor the average death for people living past the age of twenty has increased significantly since 1800. The average age of death increased steadily until 1950, but this was due to an improved childhood mortality rate. . . . For someone reaching sixty years of age, there is only a one-year difference in life expectancy between the eighteenth century and today" [4]—despite modern medical wonders of recent years.

Well over 1,000,000 people a year die of heart diseases. Dr. Wilfrid Shute quotes Dr. Paul Dudley White, the eminent heart specialist of Massachusetts General Hospital in Boston, as writing: "When I graduated from medical school in 1911, I had never heard of coronary thrombosis, which is one of the chief threats to life in the United States and Canada today—an astonishing development in one's own lifetime! There can be no doubt but that coronary heart disease has reached epidemic proportions in the United States, where it is now responsible for more than fifty percent of all deaths." [5]

The World Health Organization (WHO) of the United Nations has spent twenty-five years in a world-wide endeavor to furnish pure water, eradicate disease-carrying insects, inoculate against disease, and teach sanitation and good nutrition. They make constant comparisons of the geographical locations of various diseases in trying to determine the causes and combat them most effectively. Certainly no group has a more comprehensive view of the people of the world and their health, and they make the profound statement that "good nutrition means good health." When asked what precautions can be taken in infancy to try to overcome the diseases of the world, they say "diet."

The United States is not a healthy nation—the fact that with a population of 200,000,000 people we spend some $80,-000,000,000 a year on medical care is evidence of this. One doctor with WHO alluded to our affluence as affecting our eating habits, and that certainly is a contributing factor. Children as well as adults can afford all the junk foods. And a sign of our affluence, as well as our nutritional ignorance, is that a shopper complains about the price of food and then loads her shopping cart with the ridiculously expensive mixes and convenience foods—foods which she could make far more nutritiously, deliciously, and inexpensively herself.

According to our Department of Health, Education, and Welfare figures, an increasing percentage of young people between the ages of seventeen and twenty-four are afflicted with various chronic conditions. Between the years of 1962 and 1967 the incidence of disease in this group climbed from 37.7 to 44.6%. Even more frightening are the projections which indicate that if the recent rate continues, all of our seventeen to twenty-four-year-olds will be afflicted with one or more chronic ailments by the turn of the century!

Our nation is far from healthy, and it is getting worse. Tranquilizers are doled out to 40% of our population and each year we have a higher incidence of cancer. Dr. Cheraskin, well known in the fields of preventive medicine and dentistry, believes the saying that "Health is the fastest growing failure in America." If we do not want to pass on our ills to our children and grandchildren, we must heed the nutritional studies which show that healthy nations eat healthful foods.

Our National Diet

We eat more candy than eggs; we eat more sugar than vegetables, fruits, and eggs put together; we drink more soft drinks than milk; and beginning in 1971 we started eating more processed foods than fresh. We do not have to be nutritionists to know that this is a downhill race we are in; unless we make a drastic change, we are leading our children and grandchildren to a higher incidence of degenerative diseases than our present deplorable rate.

I think our problem is that we have not added up our diet. We think a little sugar here and there, a soft drink now and then, a little additive to a food, and "enriched" flour cannot hurt. But that is not realistic. Refined foods, sugar, and additives are in almost everything we eat, and we do not figure our actual milk intake against the soft drinks we consume and let our children consume.

All our children have to do is eat what we give them and watch us, and they will have poor eating habits. Added to this, they have $75,000,000 worth of television advertisements enticing them with promises of gimmicks and sugar. In fact, there are now more than thirty-seven kinds of sugar-coated tooth decayers—all claiming to be nutritious—from which to choose on the cereal shelf. When you add to this what we do *not* give our children—whole-grain breads and cereals, properly cooked meats and vegetables, wholesome drinks and desserts which growing children need badly, along with vitamin and mineral supplements—we should not wonder at the ills they develop. They inherit weaknesses from us through several generations of poor nutrition, and then we let them add new ones of their own. And we talk about bringing up our children in a good Christian home! What we mean is that we have looked after two-thirds of our responsibility to the best of our ability. But we have left out the other third—an abundance of God's provisions for the bodies of which we are stewards.

There are volumes of evidence that our diet is a national disaster. And that diet is getting worse.

PART 2

The Alteration of Food

Why do you spend your money for that which is not bread,
and your labor for that which does not satisfy?
Isaiah 55:2, RSV

Chapter 3

Flour, Rice, Sugar

To understand why our diet is a national disaster and what you and I can do to overcome it, we must first understand what has happened to much of the food we eat. It is depleted and adulterated in many ways and all for the convenience and profit of industry. Major ways in which our foods are altered are by milling flour, polishing rice, and refining sugar.

Flour

A century ago the high-speed roller mill came into existence. The process made milling highly profitable; it enabled millers to ship flour, baked goods, cereals, and other products to any part of the world because they did not spoil. They did not spoil because the processing successfully removed the germ containing almost all the minerals and vitamins, approximately twenty known beneficial elements, which make flour the staff of life. Isn't it interesting that God created the germ with life-giving properties and this is exactly the part man removed? Bugs, of course, are not interested in grain from which life has been removed—only man would be so foolish. Fortunately these elements, and the grain itself, are still available to us. We simply have to know where.

Although the fact that refined bread is not as nutritious as whole-grain bread has been known for generations, it is altogether possible that early manufacturers did not realize to what extent they were robbing consumers of essential nutritional elements. The story today, however, is entirely different. Tremendous research has been done over a long period of time by independent, unbiased scientists and research foundations. They have turned up massive evidence of the nutritional deficiencies of refined flour.

Today, refined flour not only has the germ removed, but an assortment of twenty different chemicals and bleaching agents are used to further alter the original food value of flour, breads, cereals, pastas, cakes, and mixes we eat today. Pitifully few vitamins and minerals are replaced, but industry has conjured up such adjectives as "enriched" and "fortified" to give the impression that all are replaced. On top of this deception, the manufacturer runs advertisements telling the public how healthful his product is and implying that athletes are strong because they eat it. When we eat refined food, we are getting only a fraction of the benefits the Great Physician prescribed for us.

By eating refined flour and sugar, we not only deprive ourselves of superior nutrition, but of fiber, which is vital to the proper functioning of our systems. This realization is not new; it dates back to Hippocrates in 400 B.C. and has been supported by certain doctors and nutritionists ever since.

What is new is that medical doctors have recently turned up their own evidence corroborating the fact that fiber is vital to health. Medical research has revealed that the lack of fiber contributes to major diseases of Western man: diverticular disease, polyps, appendicitis, cancer of the large intestine, peptic ulcer, gall-bladder disease, and obesity. The lack of fiber, because it causes sluggish circulation, also contributes to the development of hemorrhoids, varicose veins, and heart disease.

Dr. Miles Robinson reports in *Executive Health* that Surgeon-Captain Thomas L. Cleave, formerly director at the Institute of Naval Medicine in England, demonstrated as long ago as 1956 that the basic cause of many diseases could be the lack of roughage in the diet.[1] He pointed out that the refining of carbohydrates, particularly flour and sugar, inflicted *concentrat-*

ed products on the body which the body was never designed to handle.

Ninety percent of the 11,000 items on the shelves of the average supermarket have been virtually stripped of roughage through refining and manufacturing. Dr. Cleave, in his latest book,[2] explains that the removal of roughage from our food greatly slows the passage of food through the intestines which produces diverticular disease and is a strong factor in cancer of the colon. Dr. David Reuben informs us that over 99,000 new cases of colon and rectal cancer occur in our nation each year, resulting in more than 49,000 deaths. This means that on an average someone develops this form of cancer every five minutes, and every ten minutes someone dies from it.[3]

Dr. Cleave further explains that the relatively stagnant accumulation of feces presses on the great pelvic veins; this raises the pressure in the veins and slows the flow of blood. The results can include hemorrhoids, varicose veins, and thrombosis.

In addition, refined foods do not satiate the system as do natural foods. Therefore, the over-consumption of food and obesity occur. Dr. Robinson explains that adding sugar to the diet of both men and animals will raise blood cholesterol, but adding fiber will lower it. "Thus," Dr. Cleave concludes, "all these diseases and others, although appearing to be *separate* diseases, become only the manifestations of a *master disease*, consisting of refined carbohydrates, showing up in the various digestive, circulatory and other bodily systems." [4]

Dr. Denis Burkitt, of the British government's Medical Research Council, has followed up on Dr. Cleave's "brilliant conception," as he terms it, and has generated widespread interest in the subject. Many of us have been alerted through the syndicated news columns of Dr. T. R. Van Dellen and Dr. Jean Mayer,[5] who quote Dr. Burkitt. Dr. Burkitt cites the study which was made of 4000 consecutive autopsies in Uganda where unrefined cereal is a staple. Not one case of diverticular disease was found. Yet, when Africans moved into cities and adopted European ways of life, they ate less fiber and colonic lesions began to occur among them. Dr. Reuben states that nearly 1,000,000,000 men and women around the world are virtually immune to these diseases. It has been said that these particular diseases which plague the Western world today were unknown to our ancestors through thousands of generations. So returning to natural food, real food, with its splendid nutrition, its fiber, and its balanced content of natural sugar is hardly a fad.

There has been, as Dr. Robinson contends, "a shallow and inadequate view of the importance of fiber deficiency in the diseases of Western man." Adding a teaspoon or so of bran to the daily diet, which many doctors now prescribe, is better than none, but it certainly does not compensate for the nutritional inadequacy of our diet. Food which retains its full nutritional value as well as its fiber is essential to the treatment of the major diseases of the Western world.

Refined flour, then, stripped as it is of both nutrients and fiber, is hardly the staff of life. To the contrary, it apparently is the cause of more problems than most of us could have imagined. Jesus said, "I am the bread of life" (John 6:35). Obviously He was not referring to that soft, white, depleted substance the majority of Christians eat today and use to feed their families, their friends, and the poor. Therefore, it is important for us to market with a new set of eyes and new values—eyes which read all labels and values based on God's normal and wise provisions for us.

When we market for breads and cereals, we have a distinct choice to make. For instance, do we want food, such as Breakfast Squares, with the following ingredients (listed in order of their predominance): "Sugar, Shortening, Water, Enriched Flour (bleached), Dried Milk Protein, Isolated Soy Protein, Peanut Butter, Soy Protein Concentrate, Glycerine, Refiners Syrup, Mono and Diglycerides, Corn Starch, Dried Egg Whites, Salt, Artificial and Natural Flavoring, Leavening, Dextrose, Calcium Carbonate, Sodium Caseinate, Calcium Phosphate, Soy Lecithin, Calcium Sulfate, Cocoa, Vitamin A, Vitamin E, Gum Arabic, Niacin, Iron, B_6, Riboflavin, Thiamin, Vitamin D, Potassium Iodide, Vitamin B_{12}, Freshness preserved with Sodium Propionate, BHA, BHT, and Citric Acid in Propylene Glycol and Propyl Gallate"? Or do we want the staff of life—100% whole grain, 100% natural flavor, 100% nutritious, 100% chemical free, and 100% delicious?

The supermarket shelves are loaded with concoctions containing altered foods such as milled corn, sugar, oat flour, wheat flour (refined), rice (polished), salt, defatted wheat germ, malt syrup, certified colors, vitamin A, sodium ascorbate, ascorbic acid, B_1, B_2, E, B_6, folic acid, iron, BHA and BHT; and we fool ourselves into believing what the advertisements say—that we are getting all of the mentioned vitamins we need for the entire day. The next time you go marketing for cereal, remember the staff of life and don't be misled by the list of vitamins. Do not be robbed financially or nutritionally.

The few vitamins that are added to refined cereals simply play on the nutritional illiteracy of the nation and bring inordinate profits. To illustrate the point, Ray Wolfe tells us in his article "Enriched Food—Less Nutrition at Higher Cost"[6] that one brand of wheat flakes overcharges the consumer 3,000%. He says that Michael Jacobson, a Ph.D. in microbiology from Massachusetts Institute of Technology and a food additives expert, told the Consumer Subcommittee of the Senate Commerce Committee that Americans are being overcharged for foods that are packaged and advertised to be fortified. Dr. Jacobson showed that the only differences between 12-ounce boxes of Wheaties and Total were the amounts of fortified vitamins and the prices. He told the subcommittee that the wholesale cost of the added vitamins in a 12-ounce box of Total was only 0.6 of a cent, and the consumer paid 18 cents for it. This, Dr. Jacobson noted, was apparently what Hoffman-LaRoche meant in its ad for manufacturers: "We can show you why it pays to fortify." Ray Wolfe says that "the only things that become enriched are the pockets of the manufacturers."

By the same token, the next time you reach for enriched bread among the dozens of loaves on the supermarket shelf, remind yourself that you are depriving yourself and those you feed of a goodly percentage of protein, as well as other important elements. For instance, the refining of wheat removes 71% of the phosphorus, 85% of the magnesium, 77% of the potassium, and 78% of the sodium. Dr. Miles H. Robinson tells us that 76% of the iron is removed; it is replaced, but in a form which is poorly absorbed. Besides this, Dr. Henry A. Schroeder of Dartmouth Medical School says that milling removes the following percentages of essential minerals: "40% of the chromium, 86% of the manganese, 89% of the cobalt, 68% of the copper, 78% of the zinc, 48% of the molybdenum, and none of these are replaced by 'enrichment' and 'fortification.' " Besides this, you are getting an assortment of chemicals you would do well to avoid. We read that chemicals are added to prolong shelf life and assure freshness. Ross Hume Hall informs us, however, that we are not told that most are added solely to facilitate manufacturing. So, as Dr. Richard Heumer, of the Molecular Disease Institute, says, "Go to nature right now. There are all the life factors we do know about as well as the life factors we don't know about." Moreover, as we are told by Dr. Hall, "government agencies designed to guard the safety and wholesomeness of the nation's food ... do not comprehend the effects of transformed technology." And, he asks, "is there anyone who is now prepared to start examining the diverse effects of chemical manipulation of wheat molecules?" His admonition is, "Eat chemical bread at your own risk." [7]

If we are concerned about the cost of natural cereals in comparison to processed varieties, it is good to know that they run 69 to 79 cents a pound, while average cereal made of depleted grains, sugar, and chemicals run around 90 cents a pound. Then, of course, you can make your own granola at home for considerably less than the natural packaged cereals.

Today there is a wide selection of whole-grain cereals, including good old-fashioned oatmeal which may be eaten cold or cooked or used in baking. (Do not buy the quick-cooking oatmeal.) Irish and Scotch oatmeals are also to be found in many supermarkets.

Natural cereals are now appearing in the supermarket, but some are not completely natural. Check the labels. The natural cereals now produced by Pet Incorporated, Colgate-Palmolive, Quaker Oats, General Mills, and Kellogg, whose labels show natural cereals, no additives, and no preservatives, all have sugar added. Four of these products list sugar as the second ingredient which indicates that there is a considerable quantity. There is a wide variety of nutritious breads, some of which are to be found in supermarkets, but check labels to see there are no additives or sugar.

Many health food stores carry an excellent selection of whole-grain breads, including muffins, crackers, and cookies. Baking bread at home is coming back into vogue, and if that interests you, you will delight in the many recipes for it in natural food cookbooks. And you can make twice as many loaves of whole-wheat bread for close to half the cost of one loaf of "enriched." When one becomes used to eating foods made of whole-grain flours, refined flour seems monotonous, if not insipid, in contrast. So, whether you buy whole-grain products or bake them, you are in for a variety of taste treats.

To substitute nutritious and flavorful whole-grain flours for white flour, there is a general rule which can be applied. Except for whole-wheat flour, which seems to work out for me in the same proportions as refined flour, other whole-grain flours may vary some. The general rule is:

> ¾ cup whole-grain flour
> 1 tablespoon less oil
> 1 to 2 tablespoons more liquid
> for 1 cup white flour
> depending upon desired con-
> sistency
> or
> ½ cup soy flour and ½ cup
> wheat germ (and 1 table-
> spoon brewer's yeast,
> optional)

bearing in mind that whole-grain flours, like refined flour, may vary within themselves and require more or less moisture in baking. This is controlled by adding the amount of flour necessary for the desired consistency.

For thickening agents, it is not necessary to use white flour at all. In fact, the whole-grain flours lend much more interesting flavors. For instance, I use brown rice flour for lamb gravy and oat, soy, or whole-wheat flours for cream sauces. Other thickening agents besides whole-grain flours are cornstarch, potato flour, tapioca starch, arrowroot, and egg yolks. When baking with soy flour, lower the oven temperature by 25 degrees because soy flour browns more quickly. For additional nutrition, to 1 cup whole-wheat flour, add 1 tablespoon each brewer's yeast, soy flour, and wheat germ.

Whole-grain flours may be combined in any proportions desired—whole wheat, buckwheat, rye, millet, brown rice, corn, oat, barley, and soy. Some wheat or rye flours are often used in a combination of flours because of their gluten which gives dough its elasticity. However, gluten flour can be added to other flours if desired.

The Rodale Cookbook recommends the combination of oat and barley flour for pie crust and oat and soy flour to coat baked chicken.

Whole-grain breads, cakes, muffins, and such are coarser, firmer, more crumbly than the soft, spongy white bakery products they replace in your diet, but they have more flavor and are also more satisfying. Lighter products can be made by sifting whole-wheat flour, even whole-wheat pastry flour (which you do not ordinarily do), but return those good siftings to your bag of flour to be used later in breads, pancakes, and such. If a delicate texture is needed for occasional special pastries, combine whole-grain sifted pastry flour with sifted unbleached flour, half and half. Unbleached flour has nothing to offer above white flour except that it has missed one depleting process—bleaching. It does have all the drawbacks of refining and additives so we should not use it often or we will be losing some nutrition.

Whole-grain flours should be refrigerated. I keep the two I use most often in large refrigerator jars, and I buy five or six other varieties in small bags. I stand them up in a square baking tin and fold over the tops of the small bags with masking tape which makes them easy to use.

To illustrate the fun we have had with natural foods in our family, I will share a few of our family recipes.

My father's pancakes were made of a combination of from five to seven whole-grain flours. With a little meat and a little honey or 100% maple syrup, they were a great way to start the day.

Father's Whole-Grain Pancakes,
Waffles, or Muffins

3 eggs, separate into mixing bowls
2 tablespoons each:
    whole-wheat flour
    brown rice flour
    millet flour
    graham flour
    rye flour
    cornmeal

1 teaspoon salt
1 cup buttermilk
2 tablespoons oil
¾ teaspoon tartrate baking powder

Mix the flours, cornmeal, and salt together in a bowl. Beat the egg yolks and beat in the buttermilk and oil. Beat egg whites almost stiff, add the baking powder, and beat until it forms creamy peaks. Fold egg yolk mixture into egg whites and bake on heavy skillet or griddle on which oil has been poured, heated, and the excess poured off. The batter is very puffy and light; spread it a little with a spoon to form the size pancake desired.

For pancakes only, the eggs need not be beaten separately if time does not allow. In this case, all ingredients are combined and stirred well or put in a blender.

Our son, Bob, created his own crepe recipe which is ideal for brunch, lunch, or supper. They are extra special because Bob grinds his own grain for his flour just prior to putting the recipe together.

Bob's Crepes

¾ cup whole-wheat flour
3 eggs
1½ cups milk
½ teaspoon salt
1 tablespoon oil

Combine in blender and blend well or beat together with wire whisk. Oil a crepe pan (or small skillet). Pour only enough batter in to cover the bottom, turning the pan to make crepe as thin as possible. Cook briefly on both sides; stack one on another and keep warm. When all crepes are cooked, fill with creamed chicken or shredded pot roast and roll up. Crepes may also be served with butter and pure maple syrup or honey.

To recapture the life that manufacturers have taken out of wheat, buy the wheat germ itself.

Wheat Germ and Wheat Germ Oil

Wheat germ is the vital part or source of new growth in each wheat kernel. It is a rich source of protein, it is rich in all the vitamins of the B complex, and it is one of the best natural sources of vitamin E. It contains concentrated minerals: iron, phosphorus, and vitamin A. Wheat germ oil is high in E but does not contain the B complex vitamins of the wheat germ. Thomas K. Cureton Jr., director of the Physical Fitness Institute of the University of Illinois, found wheat germ oil beneficial in fighting fatigue and promoting endurance. Dr. Cureton believes that middle-aged men may reverse their age characteristics from ten to fifteen years by taking mild exercise combined with 1½ teaspoons of wheat germ oil daily. Many athletes take wheat germ oil. (As do our dogs! Only we give them 1 tablespoon daily.)

How to use: Wheat germ should be purchased in vacuum-packed containers and, once opened, should be kept tightly closed and refrigerated. It may be sprinkled over cereals or used as a cereal itself. It may be sprinkled over fruit, soup, salad, or yogurt. It may be added to cooked foods and used as "breading" for baked foods, and it may be added to milk drinks. It may also be added (1½ teaspoons per cup) to unbleached flour to fortify it.

Wheat germ oil may be taken from the bottle or added to salad dressing, one-fourth wheat germ oil to three-fourths salad oil. It should be kept in a dark bottle, tightly closed and refrigerated. It should be used up quickly as it becomes rancid.

Rice

Rice in its natural state, which is brown rice, is another food that not only contains valuable properties which have sustained people for generations in many parts of the world, but is also delightfully flavorful as well. However, in its polished state, which is the white rice with which we are most familiar, it has suffered the same depletions as the other refined grains. After the Far East adopted polished rice, they paid a certain price; beriberi is the well-known result. Interestingly enough, rice polishings are used in its cure. Although rice is not the basis of our meals, as it is in the Orient, we have been deprived.

Catharyn Elwood tells us in her book, *Feel Like A Million,* that brown rice, although listed as a carbohydrate, has excellent protein value with all eight essential amino acids well-proportioned. She also explains that polishing and refining natural brown rice robs it of its antineuritic factor (the B complex vitamins) as well as most of the essential proteins and minerals.[8]

Brown rice tastes so much better than white, polished rice that one wonders how the white was ever accepted. However, it does take a little more cooking time than white rice.

Method for Cooking Brown Rice

1 cup uncooked brown rice, rinsed in cold water
2½ cups water
½ teaspoon sea salt

Place all ingredients in a saucepan. Cover tightly and bring to a boil. Turn down heat and simmer for 40 minutes or until all the water is absorbed. The rice should be tender and separated.

Rice Polish

Rice polish is the nutritious bran layer which has been removed to produce white rice. It is high in minerals and may be added to cooked cereals, baked dishes, protein drinks, and to other flours in baking. It can be used in proportions as high as half and half to other flours. Rice polish is available in health food stores.

Wild Rice

Wild rice has about twice as much protein content as natural brown rice, according to Catharyn Elwood, and is richer in the B complex vitamins. It is expensive, but it can be purchased mixed with brown rice which cuts the cost down and makes a delicious dish. Wild rice can be cooked like brown rice. However, there is another method for cooking it alone.

Method for Cooking Wild Rice

3 cups boiling water or stock (chicken or beef)
1½ cups wild rice, rinsed in cold water

Place the rice in a pot, pour boiling water or stock over it and stir. Cover tightly and let stand overnight to absorb the liquid. Reheat to serve.

Sugar

Another abuse perpetrated by man is the addition of sugar to almost every product, including some formulas and baby foods. If this sounds like an exaggeration, and indeed it did to me, you have only to read the labels on all the canned, packaged, and frozen foods on the market. Some may even be surprised at what they find on their own kitchen shelves and in their freezers. I have heard Dr. Carlton Fredericks, the nutritionist, say that on an average we eat the equivalent of ⅓ teaspoon of sugar every half hour, twenty-four hours a day, seven days a week. The first reaction most people have is to deny this because they do not suspect all the hidden sugar they eat which has been added to almost every bottled, packaged, canned, and frozen food. It is even added to all sorts of medicinal preparations, including antacids, where its presence does not have to appear on the label.

Dr. Fredericks says that the natural sugars in food run 13% to 14%, the form in which we are intended to consume them. Refined sugar is not like natural sugar; it is 100% sugar, and we eat from 104 to 170 pounds of it a year. For instance, we swallow 5 ounces of sugar without a thought in many of our ordinary dishes. We would have to eat approximately 2½ pounds of sugar beets or 20 apples to consume the same amount in natural form. Also, there is a difference in the sugars. In *Sugar Blues,* William Dufty defines for us the difference in sugars:

> *Glucose* is a sugar found usually with other sugars, in fruits and vegetables. It is a key material in the metabolism of all plants and animals. Many of our principal foods are converted into *glucose* in our bodies. Glucose is always present in our bloodstream, and it is often called blood sugar.
> *Fructose* is fruit sugar.
> *Maltose* is malt sugar.
> *Lactose* is milk sugar.
> *Sucrose* is refined sugar made from the sugar cane and sugar beet.[9]

Glucose has always been an essential element in the human bloodstream. Sucrose addiction is something new in the history of the human animal.

Through the years our children have been educated to

sugar from the cradle up, making us a sugar-oriented nation. An example of how children are encouraged to eat sugar is one with which we are familiar. On October 28, 1972, a survey was made by a group called Action for Children's Television. They reported that in Boston alone on that day between the hours of 7:00 A.M. and 2:00 P.M. there were sixty-seven television commercials for sweetly flavored products. In January, 1976, F. Earle Barcus, a professor at Boston University's School of Public Communications, reported on a study of commercials which showed that they interrupt children's television programs about once every 2.9 minutes. Half of these commercials are for sugar cereals, candies, and sweets.[10]

Daniel Henninger wrote an article for the *National Observer* (October 6, 1973) entitled "Soured on Sugar" which dealt with sugared cereals, zeroing in on General Mills' latest product, "Mr. Wonderful Surprize . . . Only Cereal with a Creamy Chocolate-flavor Filling." Jim Hightower said that "The big surprise, in addition to the toy inside the box, is that the contents are 30% sugar, 14% fat, and it costs $1.40 a pound." [11]

Mr. Henninger informs us that $2,000,000,000 are spent annually repairing decayed teeth, and that if all the teeth that need filling were repaired, we would spend about $8,000,000,-000 a year. He says that the cereal manufacturers' excuse for adding sugar is to make children eat their vitamins (a few of which they have added to the cereal). Needless to say, throwing in a few vitamins does not overcome the sugar. Mr. Henninger's conclusion is that "The cereal men ought to withdraw their breakfast gooeys and let the kids suffer through a little sugar withdrawal."

The Federation of Homemakers in Washington warns us to look out for sugared cereals unless we want to serve our family a food that is more candy than cereal. They report that three of General Mills' cereals contain between 30% to 50% sugar. Dr. Jean Mayer contends that cereals containing more than 50% sugar should be labeled "imitation cereal" or "cereal confection" and should be sold in the candy section. He also says that the FDA refuses to consider percentage in labeling, claiming that consumers can "get the picture of content from listing ingredients according to predominance." [12]

The sugar industry issues literature on its behalf from

Sugar Information, Inc., called "An Easy-to-Swallow Guide to Good Nutrition," which bears out Mr. Henninger's statement. It maintains that "In addition to helping satisfy the strong human demand for sweet tasting food, sugar makes other foods more pleasing—on grapefruit, for example, it takes away sourness; stirred into chocolate it sets off bitterness." [13] The "strong human demand," needless to say, has been generated through the years of sugar's overuse. The association says that our sugar consumption has not changed in forty years. However, they leave out the information that during the one hundred years prior to that it climbed from approximately 5 pounds per person per year consumption to 105 and upwards to as much as 175. And the sugar industry boasts a delivery of well over 7,000,000 tons of sugar a year to the food industry. This is the sugar industry's idea of "good nutrition." Furthermore, the Sugar Association is a billion-dollar industry which lobbies in Washington and influences government decisions.

I am happy to say that there is a growing nucleus of dentists who have a knowledge of nutrition and supplements as well as the latest developments in oral hygiene. These men, in their dedication to preventive dentistry, are conscientiously endeavoring to instruct their patients how to maintain good teeth and healthy gums. My dentist tells me that he attributes much of this constructive advance in preventive dentistry to Dr. Emanuel Cheraskin, who has degrees both in medicine and dentistry, is professor and chairman of the Department of Oral Medicine at the University of Alabama, and is an author and lecturer. He speaks to many dental groups, and we can hope that he speaks to an increasing number so that more dentists will have the opportunity to learn about preventive dentistry. According to the Colgate Company's television advertisements, the average American child between the ages of five and fifteen has eleven cavities!

We have thousands upon thousands of dentists: orthodontists to reform our dental arches and realign our teeth; regular dentists to drill for decay and fill the holes to the tune of $40,000,000 a year in gold alone; and extractionists to take care of the impossible tooth or gum conditions. If we did not spend the $4,000,000,000 a year we do on dental care in our country, I venture to say that the revolting condition of the mouths of most of us would remind us moment by moment that something is drastically wrong with our diet.

Tooth decay is prevalent when sugar intake is high and drops dramatically when sugar intake is drastically reduced. James Trager corroborates this in *The Foodbook,* speaking of England whose sugar intake is comparable to ours. The record shows that there was a sharp decline in tooth decay during World War II when sugar was rationed in England.[14]

Dr. John Yudkin, a physician and a biochemist, currently Professor of Nutrition Emeritus at London University in England and author of the book *Sweet and Dangerous,* amassed a formidable amount of information to demonstrate his premise that sugar is an extremely harmful food. Dr. Yudkin's research shows that sugar is probably the leading cause of such disorders as hardening of the arteries, heart attacks,[15] diabetes,[16] gout,[17] indigestion,[18] ulcers,[19] poor eyesight, unhealthy skin, and tooth decay.[20] He says that sugar irritates the lining of the upper alimentary canal—the esophagus, stomach, and duodenum.[21] He says that there is no excuse for an obese nation not to cut down its consumption of sugar; sugar has calories and no nutrients.[22]

It is illuminating to learn from Dr. Yudkin's book that, not overlooking other factors, sugar is by far the worse contributor to coronary ills. He tells us that the rise in coronary deaths in Britain closely followed the rise in the consumption of sugar.[23] Among other examples, Dr. Yudkin cites the research done in Africa, Israel, and St. Helena.

In South Africa the black population had almost no coronary disease, while the white and Indian population had as much as did the white population of America, Western Europe, and Australasia. Now, however, heart disease is starting to occur in the black population where sugar consumption has become increasingly higher. The rise in heart disease fits the figures for the consumption of sugar.[24]

Dr. Yudkin tells us that in Israel, Dr. A. M. Cohen of Jerusalem found that recently arrived immigrants from the Yemen had little coronary disease, though the disease was common among Yemenites who had immigrated twenty years or so earlier. Of special significance is that their diet had not only been low in sugar but quite high in animal fats and butter, but when they arrived in Israel, they began to adopt the usual high sugar diet of the country.[25]

In St. Helena a special study turned up further evidence which pointed to sugar as the cause of coronary disease common among the islanders. They eat less fat than Americans or the British, they smoke much less than Westerners, and they get plenty of exercise. St. Helena is extremely hilly and there is little mechanical transport. The only reasonable cause of their high prevalence of coronary disease, the study concludes, is their high sugar consumption; it is around 100 pounds per year per person.[26]

Dr. Yudkin contends that if a fraction of what is already known about the effects of sugar were to be revealed as pertaining to any other material used as a food additive, the material would be promptly banned.[27]

Robert Rodale, in an article in which he quotes a number of the outstanding researchers on trace minerals, touches upon yet another deleterious effect of sugar. "White sugar has not only been stripped of trace elements, but has the terrible ability to drain trace element resources from other foods in an average diet." This is of special significance since we are hearing a great deal more about how vital trace minerals are to our physical and mental health.

In view of the new stream of information coming to us on the case against sugar, I have no doubt that many will be reconsidering their use of it. I find that a few of the natural food cookbooks show some dessert recipes which call for either raw sugar or brown sugar. These are not natural foods, and we may find them eliminated in revised editions. Dr. Jean Mayer says, "Both the decaying producing cariogenic and the caloric impact of sugar—white, raw, or brown—are equally devastating." We can expect the same ills of raw and brown sugar that there are with white sugar. However, there are perfectly good and nutritious substitutes if a sweetener is needed, bearing in mind that often extra sweetening is not needed.

Brown sugar is only a little less refined than white sugar so it is no great improvement, and there is no reason for using it. It can be replaced with date sugar, molasses, or honey. Raw sugar has also gone through some of the refining processes. I have heard nutritionists say that it is no better than white sugar—only dirtier.

Substitutes for sugar are honey, unsulphured molasses, fruit juices, carob powder, 100% maple syrup, and ground dates or raisins. Some recipes call for date sugar; this means ground dates. Actually, we should call refined sugar a substitute for sweetening; the natural sweeteners came first on this earth. They are excellent sweeteners and nutritious as well. However, do not overdo them. Honey is 75% sucrose and fructose, so use it sparingly.

To substitute honey in baking, the general rule is to use 2/3 cup honey plus 1/3 cup more of whatever liquid is called for in the recipe. If no liquid is called for, then add 1/3 cup more flour to make up the difference in consistency. It does take some experimenting because all recipes will not work out with this formula. If there is a problem, remember that there are innumerable recipes already worked out in natural food cookbooks. There is no problem substituting honey for corn syrup because the amount would be the same and the consistency is not changed.

The least nutritious and often most harmful part of the average American meal are desserts—not only because of the quantity of sugar consumed in them, but also the refined flour, imitation dairy products, imitation flavors and colorings, as well as a large assortment of additives. These make very undesirable foods. However, desserts can be wholly nutritious and altogether desirable—all sorts of puddings, souffles, gelatins, ice creams, and pastries made with whole-grain flours, honey, fresh milk, butter, eggs, real flavors, natural colorings, and no additives.

Our daughter, Margo, makes an easy and delicious dessert as follows:

Refrigerator Mousse Pie

¾ cup wheat germ
¾ cup granola
½ cup melted butter

Mix the above ingredients and press firmly into a 9-inch pie plate. Place in refrigerator to chill.

½ pint whipping cream
½ teaspoon Pero, Instant Cereal Beverage
    or 1 tablespoon carob powder
Dash of cinnamon

Put together in a mixing bowl and whip until stiff. Spread in pie crust. Other flavoring may be used: carob powder, vanilla, mint, nutmeg, etc.
Top whipped cream mixture with sliced peaches or other fresh fruit.

Why spend your money on foodstuffs that don't give you strength? Why pay for groceries that don't do you any good? (Isa. 55:2, Living Bible).

Could we have any clearer directive for stewardship in the food we buy?

Chapter 4

Additives

Statements to the effect that additives have been used since time immemorial and, therefore, must be accepted as proven and beneficial are misleading. Indeed salt, herbs, spices, vinegar, and honey have been used through the ages to enhance, color, flavor, texture, and preserve food. For instance, when I was in India I found that their curries were concocted because spices preserved food and, of course, refrigeration came scores of years after the native dishes had been established. We found the curries in the north of India hotter than those in the South—the hotter the country, the hotter the curry. There are hundreds of harmless, even healthful additives in use today both by industry and the innovative cook at home. However, there are those in use today which have been proven potentially harmful or which have not been adequately tested and which other nations have banned. Many additives are complex chemicals or synthetic chemicals, and we are learning we should avoid many completely.

Why Are Additives Used?

Dr. Jacqueline Verrett, a research scientist with the Food and Drug Administration for fifteen years, has co-authored a book with Jean Carper entitled *Eating May Be Hazardous to Your Health.* The book corroborates what other research scientists have been saying: industry's use of many additives is not in the interest of the nation's nutritional needs but for increased sales and profits to themselves. There is no question that the increased use of chemicals has brought a bonanza to the food industry and that "The chemical companies and foodmakers (which are fast becoming indistinguishable) are interlocked in a mutually profitable venture with no end in sight." [1] They go on to explain that synthetic chemicals are much cheaper substitutes for flavors and colors than real fruits and vegetables, and that the profit on synthetic foods formulated from chemicals is enormous.

Additives do several things: they lengthen shelf life, they make processed foods and low-grade ingredients more palatable and eye-appealing, they prevent spoilage, and, according to Dr. Verrett, they mask deterioration. Dr. Michael Jacobson, in his book *Eater's Digest,* says, "At least in the short run, it is more profitable for a company to advocate adding vitamins (which it happens to produce) to low-grade food than to tackle the nutritional problem at its roots by helping malnourished people get better jobs and more money so they can buy more nutritious food." [2] Additives allow the manufacturer to put less of the natural ingredient into his product. Ralph Nader, in his foreword to *The Chemical Feast* (a thoroughly documented study), says that "Making food appear what it is not is an integral part of the $125 billion food industry. The deception ranges from surface packaging to the integrity of the food products' quality to the very shaping of food tastes." [3] The misuse of modern chemistry is one means of deception. When we substitute the unreal for the real, we eat inferior food. We deceive our intellects but not our constitutions.

How Many Additives We Consume

Dr. Roger Williams pointed out in his book *Nutrition Against Disease,* quoting the August 16, 1969, issue of the *Lancet,* a prominent British medical journal: "On the average one consumes in the course of a year about three pounds of chemicals that are not normal constituents of food. Some of these— preservatives, coloring agents, sweeteners—are deliberately added to food while others, such as insecticides and antibiotics, may get in there unintentionally." [4] Dr. Williams' book came out in 1971; the amount of chemical additives we consume annually has increased steadily ever since. Dr. Jacobson said that in 1972 we in the United States were eating approximately five pounds of these chemicals and that our foods contained $485,000,000 worth of several thousand additives. In 1974, Dr. E. Cheraskin told us that we were eating ten pounds of additives other than sugar, salt, corn syrup, and dextrose. Dr. Verrett says that industry representatives predict that by 1980 the sales of food additives will reach $765,000,000—a 50% jump. She describes such a "chemical feast" as a collective last supper, for we have no idea of the cumulative effect on living tissue, especially after years of consumption.

A knowledge of the quantity of additives we consume comes as a shock to many of us. With this realization it is also essential to understand that, as Dr. Carlton Fredericks explains it, "The vast majority of food additives have no counterpart in nature, therefore are not automatically compatible with the body as manufacturers would suggest."

It is not the natural food additive manufacturers use that concerns us; it is the additive which is not compatible with the chemistry of the body. Some chemicals (and bear in mind that all foods reduce to chemicals) are naturally compatible and necessary to health while others are not. We must learn to distinguish between them to the best of our ability. And, in addition, we must also consider the fact that chemical additives may show up as "safe" by themselves in the limited and inadequate testing the food industry does, but beyond this there has been no testing whatsoever of chemical additives in combination with each other. We have only to look at the number of additives which appear on the labels of the food we eat to be alarmed.

How Can Additives Affect Us?

Beatrice Trum Hunter informs us that "some additives produce chemical changes in the food itself by altering the biological structure. Chemical food additives which produce derangements in the human system are so insidious that they do not become apparent until long after the original exposure.

Because of this, they may not even be suspected as the original instigator of the trouble." [5] She also says that many food additives interfere with the normal function of vitamins and enzymes which work together closely in the body. In her latest book on additives, Mrs. Hunter discusses in detail the intricate interrelationships, the interference with vital processes, and our individual susceptibilities which the consumption of chemical additives impose upon humans.[6] Mrs. Hunter amasses so much evidence that in examining her works alone we can see the danger which lies in our giving credence to our government's stamp of safety on chemical additives.

In *Consumer Beware,* Mrs. Hunter claims that "many chemicals, including food additives and pesticides, produce the same biological effects as atomic radiation, and are known as radiomimetic chemicals, because they mimic similar effects." [7]

How Many Additives?

There are 2,764 *classifications* of intentional food additives, 1,876 of which are from coal-tar derivatives. Dr. Verrett tells us that "coal-tar dye" is synonymous with hazard and that most of the 2,000 tons of food colors we use each year are coal-tar derivatives. The same dyes are used for clothing as for food. This is what we were told by Dr. Ben Feingold of the Kaiser Foundation Hospital at the March, 1974, conference of the International Academy of Preventive Medicine. Dr. Feingold has worked extensively in the field of additives and health, and he said that among the adverse reactions caused by additives are respiratory, skin, and gastrointestinal problems.

We do not realize how many compounds are involved in imitating flavors. An example Dr. Feingold gave was that artificial pineapple takes seventeen compounds and imitation coffee flavor takes from two to three hundred! When we read the words "artificial flavor," which, by the way, are on an unbelievable number of labels, we are apt to think they use one or two compounds, and we just assume the compounds are safe. According to many research scientists today we can no longer assume this.

Additives and Children

In regard to extremely adverse reactions of additives in children, an important report was made by Dr. Feingold, author of *Why Your Child Is Hyperactive,* to the Section on Allergy at the American Medical Association Convention. The report concerns itself with a study of hyperkinetic children. Hyperkinesis is a disorder which manifests itself in over-activity, disruptive behavior, and a short attention span which may interfere with learning abilities. Dr. Feingold's group found that by feeding hyperkinetic children a salicylate-free diet (which eliminates 80% of the food additives, including artificial flavors and colors) they could eliminate or drastically reduce the disorder in fifteen out of twenty-five children. Furthermore, by returning these additives to the diet, they could trigger a return of hyperkinesis. In his March, 1974, lecture Dr. Feingold described the average child's diet as follows:

> A cereal "loaded" with nonessential flavors and colors to entice the child. A beverage, either chocolate or other drinks, most of which are rich with many artificial flavors and colors. Pancakes made from a mix, frozen waffles dyed with tartrazine, or frozen French toast. Then the conscientious and concerned mother gives the child vitamins, usually chewable which are also loaded with additives. To cap the ironical situation, the child is given a dose of methylphenidate or amphetamine before going to school. At school, where the same ritual is continued at lunch, the child receives hot dogs, luncheon meats, ice cream, and various beverages.

After this list of additive-laden foods, Dr. Feingold goes on to say, "Is it any wonder that our children are jumping and failing to learn?" As with many health problems, there are often contributing factors besides diet to be considered and corrected at the same time; in the case of hyperkinesis, allergy is one. However, the fact remains that many qualified doctors and scientists are trying to alert us to the risks we unknowingly take when we are not informed on today's food products and what effect they can have on the body. If extreme symptoms, such as those of hyperkinesis, can be due wholly or partially to additives, we do not wonder at the reports we receive on the havoc additives play in less extreme but nonetheless disturbing behavioral problems in children. And we do not wonder that adults can be similarly affected. These additives are not real food.

How Well Are We Protected?

The disillusioning aspect is that some of the drugs, colorings, and additives which are used freely and highly defended by the producers, as well as the government, are later forced off the market because of their record of ill effects. Some bans have come about because citizen groups have brought pressure to bear or because studies in other countries have been publicized. For example, in April of 1973 the government banned the use of a dye known as Violet No. 1, which has been in use for twenty-two years. The dye has been used widely in beverages, candies, bakery goods, ice creams, sherbets, drugs, cosmetics, and meat stamping (now you recognize the dye!). The dye was banned, as was Butter Yellow before it, because of studies made by the Japanese which showed the dyes to be carcinogenic.

Another example is that some coal-tar dyes labeled safe and certified ten years ago have been removed because they have since been found unsafe. Today there are still "certified" dyes in question.

The fact that so many additives were approved at one time and later found damaging does not inspire our confidence in the safety of foods in our country. In effect, we are the guinea pigs. We need not be naive any longer. Responsible researchers are convinced that our testing must be improved. Our government's ability to turn a deaf ear to the experience and caution of other countries is also disconcerting. We permit any number of additives in our foods which are banned in Europe. One is Red No. 2, or aramanth as it is also called. Dr. Harold Rosenberg quotes a 1973 *Medical World News* report: "The Soviet Union banned the coloring on the basis of research implicating it in birth defects, impaired reproduction, and cancer in rats." But in that same year "the FDA certified for use more than 1.2 million pounds of the dye, which produces the vivid cherry hue of soft drinks and is also added to ice cream, candies, baked goods, and sausage. A popular sugar-coated cornflake is sprayed bright pink with Red No. 2 and promoted to children as an energy-packed breakfast." [8]

Dr. Verrett says that we use about $19,000,000 worth of the dye in our foods. In fact, it is almost impossible to avoid because it is used in so many foods. Many took heart in January,

1976, when it was announced that the Food and Drug Administration had finally banned Red Dye No. 2. A few days later, however, the ban was held up by a federal judge who set a hearing in Washington on the manufacturer's objections to the ban. Now, however, the ban is on again until further notice. We seem to be back on the merry-go-round with a dye whose safety, the FDA says, it has not proved.

BHT and BHA (butylated hydroxytoluene and butylated hydroxyanisole) are two more additives which some other countries ban. In our country we find them on the label of almost every processed food item "to preserve freshness." They are petroleum products. They are synthetic chemicals, antioxidants, used to retard or prevent rancidity, which allows the manufacturer to ship in quantities and the grocer to stock for long periods. They are used in numerous vegetable oils and shortenings as well as in the products containing them.

The Consumer Bulletin of October, 1961, had an article entitled "The Mystery of the Butylated Twins" because it seems they were never allowed access to the actual reports on the testing of the chemicals. Dr. Jacobson ran into difficulties also. It seems that this is a common predicament because the manufacturers run the tests on the additives—not the FDA, as many of us assume. The FDA simply examines for approval the data turned over to them in the manufacturer's petition, and it is literally held as "confidential." It is a difficult and lengthy procedure for an outside investigator to get a look at the summaries in the FDA files and, apparently, some have been defeated. It is no wonder then that we, the consumers, have been kept in ignorance so long. We owe a debt of gratitude to the determination of the investigators who are interested in the nation's health instead of industry's profits.

Beatrice Trum Hunter points out that in Rumania experiments using rats fed BHT revealed such metabolic stress that their Hygiene and Public Health Institute recommended it be banned. She says that because of other tests on various animals, BHT and BHA have been banned or restricted to a very limited use in Sweden, Britain, Australia, New Zealand, and other countries. In fact, the Food and Agriculture Department of World Health Organization of the United Nations recommended a "conditional intake limit with expert supervision and advice." [9] What is the situation in the U.S.? We find BHT and BHA in so many of our foods that we could eat it at every meal and every snack every day of the year without realizing it. Jim Hightower says, "There are thousands of people with allergies to such freshness preservatives as BHT, BHA and EDTA, but hundreds of food products contain these additives without listing them on labels." [10] Sometimes we hear from the defenders of BHT that because it is an antioxidant, it can be beneficial and has been used medically in antioxidant therapy. There are natural antioxidants, however, including vitamins C, E, and selenium. The fact is, we do not have a "conditional intake limit" of BHT and BHA, nor do we take it under "expert supervision and advice." We apparently don't always know when we are taking it, but we do know it appears on the labels of hundreds of foods on the supermarket shelf. We also know that innumerable independent researchers say that BHA and BHT should be avoided; they regard these chemicals as unsafe.

NITRATE and NITRITE (saltpeter) have been used for many years in curing meat and is found in ham, bacon, luncheon meats, canned meat and fish, as well as in frankfurters, braunschweiger, and other sausages. Industry defends its use for these two reasons: one, it kills bacteria and gives meat a reddish color; two, the fatty parts of the product look red instead of an unappetizing gray—otherwise we might not buy the product.

There has been a war waging against their use because it has been found that nitrite (contained in nitrate) is one of the most toxic chemicals in our food supply. Nitrate and nitrite have been used in apparent ignorance for many years, but one wonders how their continued use can be sanctioned with the mounting incriminating evidence against them. Their use is forbidden in Japan and Germany where they are judged as cancer-producing, and, according to Dr. Jacqueline Verrett, they are condemned by scientists, including some with the FDA, in our country as well. She cites the report made in 1972 entitled "The FDA and Nitrite." It was made by Dale Hattis, a graduate student at the Stanford School of Medicine, who had filed a freedom-of-information suit to obtain all the documents, memos, etc., of the FDA pertaining to its approval of nitrite in smoked fish. The information received revealed that the FDA had approved the use of nitrate after the agency itself, in 1948, had classified it as follows: "We regard (nitrite and nitrate) as poisonous and deleterious substances not required in the manufacture of any food subject to the jurisdiction of the Food, Drug and Cosmetic Act, and, as such, any food subject to the act and containing any quantity of these chemicals would be deemed to be adulterated under the law, regardless of labeling." [11] Dr. Verrett attributes the subsequent reverse action of the FDA to their succumbing to the pressures of economic interests.

According to Dr. Jacobson, nitrate is added to more than 7,000,000,000 pounds of meat and fish annually. Dozens of persons have died from nitrate poisoning, he says, and countless others have been incapacitated. Dr. Jacobson explains that nitrate is capable of disabling hemoglobin, the molecule in red blood cells that transports life-giving oxygen. It can also combine chemicals called secondary amines to form nitrosamines which are powerful carcinogens (substances producing or inciting cancer), teratogens (deviations from normal type of organisms), and poisons.

Dr. Verrett tells us that nitrosamines are especially interesting to scientists and especially terrifying for the human race because, unlike other carcinogens, they attack all organs and, also unlike other cancer-causing chemicals, they have produced cancer in every species of animal tested. Dr. Verrett says, "There seems to be no species resistant to their ravages, and it is the wildest kind of wishful thinking to hope that people might be." Then she quotes Dr. William Lijinsky, a prominent scientist who has been working on the problem of nitrates in foods at Oak Ridge National Laboratories since 1961, who says, " 'It is most unlikely that man would be the only resistant species.' " Dr. Verrett goes on to say that "he (Dr. Lijinsky), like some other scientists, believes that nitrosamines, because of their incredible versatility in inciting cancer, may be the key to an explanation of the mass production of cancer in seemingly dissimilar populations. In other words, nitrosamines may be a common factor in cancer that has been haunting us all for years."

"Remember, even though the amount of nitrosamines might be exceedingly small, there is no guarantee that it might not be harmful because a 'no-effect' level for nitrosamines has never been established in animal studies." [12] In regard to hot dogs, bacon, bologna, and smoked fish, Dr. Lijinsky says, "In my opinion nitrites constitute our worst cancer problem. I don't touch any of that stuff when I know nitrite has been added." [13] Reportedly, in the past year government scientists have found significant levels of nitrosamines in cooked sausage, cured pork, dried beef, and fish.

A pertinent example of the harm the additive can cause comes from a researcher at the University of California Medical Center in San Francisco who says that nitrate-induced headaches, which come from frankfurters and other cured meats, are becoming a "reasonably" common problem.

Now, more than seventeen years after the passage of the Delaney Amendment (banning carcinogenic additives to food) and more than three years after consumer groups petitioned the USDA to outlaw unnecessary use of sodium nitrite, the USDA has taken action. So far, however, it is only minimal action. Bacon is considered the worst offender among cured products because it is cooked at a high temperature, and the USDA has proposed a maximum level for nitrite in bacon. But they did not propose a minimum level, which would lead us to believe that they are less concerned with its preservative properties than its value cosmetically and as a taste enhancer. Thus, many of us will continue to avoid bacon.

Nutrition Action of January, 1976, published in Washington, D.C., informs us that there is a new product on the market called "Bakon." It comes from Sioux City, Iowa, and is made of the same cut as bacon. It is 75% meat, nitrite-free, safe, and tasty.

Some health food stores carry frozen, nitrate-free hot dogs, salami, bologna, and cured meats. For years we have been enjoying Jones Sausage, which has no additives whatsoever. I also use this as a substitute for bacon bits in tossed salad, baked potatoes, and green beans; I cook the links and slice them thin or cook the patties and mince them. Good sausage may be made at home as well.

MSG (monosodium glutamate) has come under question for several reasons. The case of the CRS (Chinese Restaurant Syndrome) sparked off research which established the relation of MSG to the varied immediate symptomatic complaints. This was so widely publicized that many of us wondered if we should continue its use. I had used it upon occasion, especially where called for in Oriental dishes. I assumed that it was the same MSG which had been used in the Orient for so many years. However, I learned from Beatrice Trum Hunter's *Consumer Beware* that the version of MSG in our country is quite different. In the Orient MSG is made from soy and seaweed; in the United States it is made from wheat or corn gluten or from sugar-beet by-products, all of which are common allergens. It is also a concentrated form of sodium which is a warning to those on low-sodium diets.

Presently what we are being told is that MSG is a disguise. Mrs. Hunter, among other documented descriptions, mentions that MSG "is known to step up indifferent and undistinguished flavor of canned meat ... it acts as a color and flavor preserver ... it prevents or retards development of warmed over off flavors that develop normally during storage ... protects flavor lost through over- or under-cooking ... and has an antioxidant effect upon hams, bacon, pork sausages, fatty fish, as well as 'acceptability of MSG in frankfurters.' " She also says that restaurants have been urged to use it "to hold flavor" and overcome "steam table fatigue" for meats.[14]

Tests made by Dr. John Olney of Washington University Medical School at St. Louis showed brain damage to baby animals who had been fed MSG. Dr. Olney believes that pregnant women should not use MSG until further data is available. And inasmuch as food producers buy 40,000,000 pounds of MSG a year, perhaps further data will be made available to us all as research continues.

I have discussed, and only briefly, three additives. My hope is that this will spur the reader to make his or her own investigation and, most importantly, to avoid as many additives as possible. Dr. Linus Pauling, in speaking on the subject of "Ageing Processes," advised people to take enough vitamin C and stay away from additives. It is certainly true that we have no way of knowing what many of these chemicals are doing to us or will do to us over a period of time, especially as research scientists say that the effects are cumulative. One thing we do know is that certain chemicals in extensive use today are not naturally compatible with our bodies; they are foreign to our natural chemistry.

How Necessary Are Additives?

Most importantly, we can ask how many additives are necessary anyway? Many additives are in foods simply for their cosmetic value—making a product more eye-appealing when it seems we could be perfectly happy with the natural appearance. For instance, Dr. Verrett informs us that for years rice has been coated with glucose and talc which contains asbestos. The Rice Millers' Association, which opposes the practice, explains that this is done to give rice a glossy appearance. The manufacturers thinks this appeals to us more than the dull look of rice, thus enhancing their sales. Obviously, like polishing rice and refining flour, this is the manufacturers' game of educating the public to altered foods—otherwise the natural product would look attractive to us.

Dr. Verrett points out that the cosmetic additive to rice has a number of drawbacks: the shiny coating conceals the true appearance and nature of the rice kernal, adds cost, and necessitates washing which causes a loss of vitamins and minerals. Moreover, asbestos produces cancer of the esophagus, the stomach, the colon, and the rectum, as discovered in asbestos plants, so a thorough washing is essential. I think if we were asked, the consensus of opinion would be that we would like to be educated back to the natural beauty and character of nature's produce.

Since it is an established fact that innumerable additives can be carcinogenic, since it has been determined by some researchers that their effect is cumulative, and since there is no such thing as a "safe" level, why do we take chances? The government continues to contend that their approved levels of additives are not carcinogenic in humans; future generations may tell the story. In the meantime, who knows the sensitivity of each body chemistry, or the present accumulation of carcinogens, or the daily intake of many foods with additives? Dr. Verrett's fifteen years of research for the FDA leads her to ask the question, "Why doesn't the FDA clean up the food supply? Why must we be subjected to so many untested or unsafe chemicals in our diet, many of which if taken in pill form could be obtained only by prescription?" [15] At any rate, these chemicals are not food at all. Why not eat pure food, real food?

A knowledge of what is happening to food products today is a matter of stewardship in a number of ways; expense is certainly one. Why should we have the expense of additives? We pay the food industry to remove good nutrients, then we pay them an excessive amount to return a fraction of the vitamins and minerals they removed, and then we pay them for the chemicals they put in to fool us in one way or another. The bread industry uses more than 60,000,000 pounds of chemicals yearly, and that comes out of the consumers' pockets.

It should be the greatest interest of our food industry to guard our internal environment, not only by putting the right things into food but by leaving the destructive or questionable things out. However, if we don't want to take chances, we must guard our internal environment ourselves. The manufacturer is concerned with shelf life, not our life. One of the latest frozen, convenience, "foodless" desserts has everything artificial in it except some skim milk. When we can serve delicious desserts made with fresh eggs, milk, cheese, and fruit, pure gelatin, natural flavors, natural colors, and natural goodness, isn't it rather foolish to sit down at the table and say, "Thank you, Lord, for the water, sugar, hydrogenated vegetable oil, nonfat dry milk, modified tapioca starch, emulsifiers (polysorbate 60, sodium stearoyl-2-lactylate, sorbitan monostearate), vanilla extract, sodium casseinate, dextrose, salt, calcium carrageenan, guar gum, with artificial color and flavor. Bless it to our lives and our lives to Thy service"? That is the label, word for word, on one of the nation's popular puddings. And this is the kind of food we ask the Lord to bless to our lives and health and to His service!

Not all these additives are dangerous, but the point is that some are complex chemicals, some are thought to need more researching, and some are known to be harmful. In any event, how much real food and honest food value are we getting? Jim Hightower points out, "There may be a need for additives, and there are many natural substances to meet that need. But there is not a need for the mass of chemicals that are poured recklessly into food at the whim of the manufacturer.... The calm willingness of food firms to experiment on American eaters is quite extraordinary." [16] Hightower thinks the burden of proof should not be on the consumers, but on the manufacturers; they should show us absolutely that a chemical is *not* dangerous and *is* essential to the manufacture and sale of a necessary food product.

How Can We Protect Ourselves?

There are three important measures to take in order to protect ourselves from the continuing and increasing use of additives: market carefully, write to manufacturers, and support constructive legislation.

We can take action to bring an end to such ignorant irresponsibility in feeding ourselves and others. We can leave the foods which have additives that are harmful or in question on the shelf. We want to avoid "food from which the essential nutrients have been stripped, either in the way it is grown, produced or processed," to quote Beatrice Trum Hunter, and we want to avoid additives. What is a food without additives? Mrs. Hunter answers that question by saying:

> This means that there will be no added preservative, color, flavor, antioxidant, emulsifier, extender, modifier, bleach acidifier, clarifier, or any of the other thousands of additives now being used in food processing. It also implies that the food has not been treated with or does not contain any residue of pesticide, hormone, antibiotic, or other chemical, drug or serum that is now commonly used in food production. Nor will the food have unintentional additives, such as transferred wax, phenol, chemical, or other substances from the wrapper or packaging material.[17]

Avoid products which show "hydrogenated" fat or oil and "hydrolyzed" protein. Avoid soft drinks—even without sugar or caffeine; they have additives and no nutritional value. Avoid convenience foods, packaged meals, and mixes. Avoid canned baby foods. Avoid everything imitation, which includes fake dairy products such as whipping cream. Remember that "textured" means synthetic.

I would add to these general suggestions for marketing a quotation from the 1963–64 *Consumer Bulletin Annual:* "Be slow to use new types of foods, or complex foods, or foods treated or preserved by new techniques. Man's digestive tract was many thousands of years in development; it cannot adapt, even in a long lifetime, to new chemical and biochemical hazards."

If we leave foods in question on the shelf, retailers and manufacturers will take note that their sales are dropping. The Christian community makes a formidable army. What we buy or do not buy can turn the tide. There are extremely informative books which give specific details of foods to avoid and foods to buy when marketing. We need definitive guidelines, and I recommend some at the end of this section.

For those who would be willing to go a step further and write manufacturers asking them to refrain from their use of questionable additives, it is well to remember that the burden of proof of the safety of additives lies with the manufacturer—everything starts there.

This, then, brings us to necessary government action for our protection. Dr. Verrett, after long years in the very midst of the situation, gives some advice on what can be done to restore to consumers their right to safe foods regardless of economic and political interests. She mentions that certain members of Congress are doing their best in presenting bills which will protect us and says that these bills should be soundly supported by the consumer so they will be passed.

Dr. Verrett bemoans the fact that distinguished scientists, much of the FDA's dissenting vitality, have left. She believes the lack of expertise is compounded by the FDA's increasingly turning toward a small clique of pro-industry scientists and away from renowned scientific authorities. However, she says there remain dedicated, competent persons in the FDA who are unhappy about many of the FDA's official decisions. These men and women, like the doctors who are becoming aware of our nation's need for good nutrition, no doubt welcome consumer awareness and support of the important bills coming before Congress.

Dr. Verrett says: "Certainly organized consumer pressure is a must—and consumers should morally and financially support groups such as Ralph Nader's Center for Study of Responsive Law and Health Research Group; Dr. Jacobson's Center for Science in the Public Interest; Jim Turner's Consumer Action for Improved Foods and Drugs; Consumers' Union, and Ruth Desmond's Federation of Homemakers, which consistently watch the activities of the FDA and USDA and bring lawsuits and other pressure against them in public interest, to get dangerous chemicals removed from the market." [18]

I depend upon the Federation of Homemakers to keep specifically informed concerning the bills being presented in Congress. They also give other important and useful information to their members through their bulletins.

Read Labels

By carefully examining labels, we can easily eliminate the many additives our families have been devouring regularly for a long time. For example, Jello, which is among the first foods given to babies and is a standard item in the average American diet, is made of:

> Sugar
> Adipic acid (for tartness)
> Sodium citrate (controls acidity)
> Fumaric acid (for tartness)
> Artificial flavor
> U.S. certified color

There is no trick at all to making gelatin desserts of pure gelatin with fresh fruits or vegetables.

Jello pudding, another American staple, is made of:

> Sugar
> Coconut
> Cornstarch
> Dextrose (corn sugar)
> Modified cornstarch
> Salt
> Calcium carrageenan (vegetable gum thickener)
> Polysorbate 60 (emulsifier for uniform dispersion
>   of milk)
> Artificial flavor
> (Note the two sugars)

It is easy to make pudding with fresh eggs, milk, fruit, carob, honey, and pure flavorings. The natural foods cookbooks have many excellent recipes for puddings, gelatin desserts, and salads; *The Natural Foods Blender Cookbook* has many innovative ideas for blender gelatin dishes.

Another example is salad dressing—why insult our stomachs with commercial dressing which costs considerably more and is full of additives? For instance, commercial Italian dressing has the same few ingredients as homemade dressing (except that the oil may be cottonseed oil) and then the following are added:

> Sugar
> Flavor (whatever that means)
> Propylene Glycol
> Alginate
> Calcium Disodium
> EDTA added as preservative

EDTA stands for ethylenediaminetetracetic acid. As one biochemist says, stay away from chemical additives with which you are not acquainted, especially those with long names. One look at what EDTA stands for makes us realize how complex these chemicals can be. Another item for our information is that the designation "pure vegetable oil" can be cottonseed oil which the *Supermarket Handbook* tells us is not grown for food and is subject to many chemical sprays. The authors warn us that "Food products derived from cotton are not fit for human consumption." [19] Salad dressings without additives are available at natural food (health food) stores. Dressings are, however, easily made at home. For example, authentic Italian dressing is made of oil, vinegar, garlic, and salt. It takes no time at all and certainly no expertise. I often make my salad dressing right on the salad, which is another easy procedure.

My Daily Dressing

> 1 tablespoon vegetable oil per person
> 1 teaspoon fresh lemon juice (1 squeeze) per person
> Sea salt and pepper
> Pinch of herbs: thyme, marjoram, basil, mint, or
>   fines herbs
> Sesame, sunflower, or pumpkin seeds, toasted

I sometimes split a garlic clove and rub the salad bowl with it. I make sure that my greens are dry; moisture prevents the oil from coating the leaves well. I first sprinkle the oil over the salad and toss it; then squeeze the lemon over it and toss. Then I add the salt, herbs, and seeds and toss it very well until each leaf is shiny. I then sprinkle a little more salt and some freshly ground pepper over the salad and toss again lightly. (I prepare whatever greens and vegetables I am using and refrigerate them in the salad bowl until I am ready to use them. I put the dressing on just before serving.)

We do not need additives in our cooking or in canning. We do not even need to use sugar. Honey is satisfactory even in jams, jellies, and pickles; it is efficient and a nutritional asset as well. There are excellent books on the subject—Rodale's *Stocking Up* is one. It covers canning, freezing, brining, storing, and so forth and it carries the attractive subtitle, *How to Preserve the Foods You Grow Naturally.*

Eating out presents a problem; additives are virtually impossible to avoid. Having been in the restaurant business myself, I know that the majority of them serve a large percentage of canned, frozen, and processed foods which contain all the additives found in the merchandise in supermarkets. Restaurants are also serving an increasing number of convenience foods—your Chicken Kiev or Chicken Cordon Bleu, and many other dishes, may have come frozen from a fancy food distributor and been heated up to fill your order. When ordering, be careful to avoid the kinds of foods which are usually loaded with chemicals. If one must eat out regularly or often, it is a good idea to know your restaurant well and learn what foods are the purest and which are made from fresh produce. Ideally, of course, you can go to a good natural foods restaurant; there are a number in our country, but we need a great many more. A few wise restaurateurs are now offering natural foods specialties on their regular menus. Hopefully, with the growing awareness of good nutrition which is coming about in our country, we will see many more restaurants offering nutritious foods, as well as many more natural foods restaurants.

Surely the Scripture which says:

> Finally, brothers, whatever
> is true, whatever
> is noble, whatever
> is right, whatever is pure, whatever
> is lovely, whatever is admirable—
> if anything is excellent or
> praiseworthy—think
> about such things (Phil. 4:8).

can be applied to what we eat and drink, as well as to other areas of our Christian life.

Chapter 5

Hydrogenation, Dairy Products,

and Cheese

Hydrogenation

"Hydrogenated" is a term we see on the labels of many jars and packages, and we are apt to think it means that the contents are well-combined in some new, wonderful way. Well, it is neither new nor wonderful. It is fifty years old, it was first devised to make soap, and it is something we are advised to avoid wherever possible. There is no problem avoiding it with the packages so marked, of which there are plenty, but it is also found in prepared foods in which there is vegetable oil or shortening, and the description of the hydrogenated (or hardened) ingredient does not have to appear. This is another good reason to avoid some prepared foods.

Hydrogenation simply means adding hydrogen to unsaturated fats (vegetable oils—which are naturally liquid) to give them the character of saturated fats (animal fats—which are naturally solid). The manufacturers of commercial shortenings such as Crisco and Spry make them by taking vegetable oils and hydrogenating them. Peanut butter which does not eventually separate is hydrogenated.

Gene Marine and Judith Van Allan, in their book *Food Pollution,* say that when margarine manufacturers claim their products to be "high in polyunsaturates," it is a relative claim. After all, margarine is made of hydrogenated vegetable oil, emulsified with milk and other additives, and its very consistency—solid—is a direct measure of how saturated it actually is. The authors further explain that there is a "serious catch" to magarine: "The parts of vegetable oils which contain these carbohydrate chains are acids—fatty acids. And it turns out that the fatty acids in vegetable oils have important functions in our metabolism—so important that some of them are now generally referred to as 'essential fatty acids.' " [1] Albert von Haller is quoted as saying that "these unsaturated fatty acids play their part in preserving the healthy state of the blood vessels and the skin, in promoting normal growth and in protecting the organism against infections. This many-sidedness of their functions points to the fact that they do not merely have a limited local significance, but that, like the vitamins, they are absolutely essential for the proper functioning of the body's metabolism as a whole." [2]

Therefore, if you wish to cut down on your cholesterol intake, instead of using margarine, blend 2/3 cup of pure creamery butter with 1/3 cup safflower oil and limit your intake by spreading it thin. Good vegetable oils, such as safflower, sesame, sunflower, soy, peanut, or a mixture, may be used in cooking wherever margarine or butter are called for in a recipe.

Mrs. Hunter believes that in light of present knowledge, official acceptance of hydrogenation is unpardonable. These seem reasons enough to make every effort to keep all hydrogenated oils, and products which contain them, out of the house. They are in widespread use for the usual reasons manufacturers give—they keep well, they are economical, they facilitate food preparation, and, of course, they bring higher profits. They are to be found in baked goods, margarine, imitation milk, non-dairy cream substitutes, peanut butter, some convenience foods, and many other products.

Dairy Products

Some of us accept non-dairy substitutes without question, and we like the idea of fat-free whipping cream substitutes. But we might think twice if we knew what we were substituting. For instance, Jim Hightower informs us that Lucky Whip is "a fabrication of Unilever's imagination, containing only water, vegetable oil, sugar and more than a dozen chemicals, for which you pay more than you would for real whipping cream."[3]

Many of us today do not know the difference between certified raw milk and pasteurized milk. The National Health Federation Bulletin describes the difference between them. Certified raw milk exceeds pasteurized milk nutritionally and requires far stricter sanitation controls. The cows used for certified raw milk are tested daily at an independent laboratory for the Certified Milk Commission, and the bacteria plate count for standard plate count is 10,000 milliliter maximum. Cows used for pasteurized milk are tested twice a month by the Health Department, and the bacteria plate count for standard plate count is 50,000 per milliliter maximum. A tuberculosis test is made every 180 days by the state veterinarian for the certified milk and annually for pasteurized milk. Employees at certified milk farms are given monthly health examinations; at pasteurized milk farms only one health examination is required, and that is at the time of employment.

Nutritionally, raw milk retains all available enzymes, protein, amino acids, fatty acids, both saturated and unsaturated, vitamins, carbohydrates, and minerals. The enzyme factor takes on new significance because it is now thought that the enzymes are important to the digestibility of milk, and it could be that this is the reason some babies cannot tolerate formulas. In pasteurizing, less than 10% of the enzymes remain. The proteins, fats, carbohydrates, and minerals are all altered (meaning loss at varying degrees of metabolic availability), and there is a vitamin loss of from 30% to 80% depending upon pasteurization temperature.

A great deal of false information has been spread about certified raw milk. It is important to know that Dr. Barnard Bellew, who has made an intensified study of certified raw milk and pasteurized milk comparisons, states unequivocally "that there has never been one documented case of infection or disease transmitted to man from certified raw milk. No other food can claim this enviable record." [4]

One of the examples Dr. Bellew gives us of the actual data

on problems with milk-borne disease is as follows:

> Suffice it to say that in 1968 70% of all milk-borne disease was from pasteurized milk products and only 30% from raw milk. Of the raw milk infections, none was from *certified* (emphasis added) raw milk, but rather, from untested family cows. All of the above could have been and should have been prevented. If all milk met certified standards, and all milk was taken as certified raw milk for supreme nutrition there would be no milk infections. Health officials should up-date this milk statistic and publish daily food infection Box Scores on disease from all foods.[5]

We learn from Dr. Bellew's article that there are three states now selling pure certified raw milk: California, New York, and Georgia. The dairies are Alta-Dena in City of Industry and Laurelwood Acres, Ripon (goat's milk), both in California, Mathis Dairy in Decatur, Georgia, and Gates Dairy in New York.

Harold Stueve, head of Alta-Dena, backed by his eleven brothers and five sisters, is credited with saving certified raw milk for our country. Dr. Bellew concludes that the rest succumbed to the terrible pressures arising from the promoters of pasteurization. The Stueves say, "We believe that God gave us food in its fullest nutritional capacity, and it is up to the people to handle it and protect it as such." [6] Dr. Bellew agrees and adds that "man has never been able to improve on certified raw milk, or any other God-given natural food."

Dr. Bellew says, "None of the big pasteurized milk interests felt comfortable in the knowledge that their production would be checked daily by the American Medical Milk Commission if they opted for certified milk." [7] This no doubt accounted for our losing a good many certified milk producers. I feel fortunate to be living in a state where I can purchase licensed raw milk. Anyone interested in having raw milk can look in the *Classified Directory* under "Dairies" for sources of raw milk; new ones are coming into existence.

Cheese

When it comes to cheese, we have the natural and the unnatural. As we know, we have all sorts of processed foods on the market; one of these is processed cheese, simply called "process cheese."

The substitute for natural cheese in one of the atrocities of this age; we suffer for it both nutritionally and gastronomically. Process cheese is made by grinding cheese of any quality and mixing in chemicals and emulsifiers.

Nikki and David Goldbeck tell us that the supposed advantage of process cheeses over natural cheeses is that "they melt and spread easily and smoothly and are thus considered more convenient. The flavor, however, never approaches the richness of natural cheese, the controlled texture is dull, and a large part of the price goes toward the purchase of chemicals." [8] Beatrice Trum Hunter notes that along with the less than desirable quality and the chemicals in process cheese, it is made quickly by heat and then aerated to increase volume. She considers that the end product scarcely deserves the classification of food.

Natural cheeses are real food and excellent food. They are high in protein and calcium and contain phosphorous, amino acids, vitamin A and some of the B vitamins which make them an important, as well as an economical, part of any meal. However, as we may have suspected, natural cheeses in America may not be as natural as we would like. Some natural cheeses have undergone the additive treatment like so many other foods, so again, labels must be scrutinized. The dairy industry has slipped by through the years without the same labeling requirements imposed upon the manufacturers of other foods; hence, all additives will not appear on the label, such as artificial coloring. Thus, white cheddar is safer to buy than the yellow-orange for this reason. However, preservatives and bleached milk must appear on the labels. (By the way, the cheese called American Cheese is never natural.)

We are enthusiastic cheese eaters in our family, and we invariably buy imported cheeses. Europeans cherish their cheeses and are anxious to keep them superior, both in flavor and texture. I should say that we do purchase un-aged cheese, such as cottage cheese and kefir cheese, from our health food store. Otherwise, we frequent cheese shops which carry imported cheeses and indulge especially in those from Denmark and Switzerland. Besides using cheese melted on toast, in soufflés and casseroles, we use it cubed in salads, grated over vegetables and soups, and we often serve an assortment with fruit for dessert.

Chapter 6

Chemicals and Drugs in Farming, Mass Production of Fruits and Vegetables, Convenience Foods

It is amusing to hear people speak of health foods and organic farming as "fads." These things are centuries old. Actually, the fads are the modern-day, ever-changing methods of farming, the raising of animals with manufactured chemicals and drugs, and the overprocessing, coloring, preserving, and sweetening of so many food products. Many of our present food products were not heard of one hundred, or fifty, or ten years ago, and many will be changed tomorrow. We have a phantasmagoria of foods. We do not know how long these modern foods and methods will last, but we do know that eating unadulterated food is as old as man and that practicing the method of natural gardening has been going on since the first gardener —a pretty long time for a fad to last! It is our responsibility to distinguish between faddism and natural, normal provision.

Gardening

As organic farmers will tell you, the organic principle amounts to simply working with nature rather than against it; when you respect the soil and take care of it, it will take care of you. Organic gardening is the accepted term to describe the raising of plants and animals without the use of manufactured and synthetic chemicals. The proponents of manufactured chemicals are quick to defend their methods by pointing out that all substances, natural or manufactured, are reduced to chemicals in the process of fertilizing. This, of course, is true but does not take away one iota from the reasons the farmers have who prefer the natural method. Just as the controversy over synthetic and natural vitamins rages, so does the dispute over what is termed "organic gardening" and gardening with manufactured chemicals. The basis for the natural in both cases is logical. The natural substances may have, and in many cases do have, other yet unidentified components which there is every reason to believe are complementary. This is the genius, the miracle, of nature. We have only scratched the surface.

Ross Hume Hall points out that no one questions the objectives of mechanical agriculture. He says:

> One objective of agricultural technology is to bypass as many of Nature's systems as possible—to simplify nature's complex cycles. Artificial fertilizers, in the opinion of agricultural technologists and scientists, eliminate the need for the complex life of the soil. To these experts, the soil is a lifeless substance whose sole function is to support the roots of the plant. The agriculturist will provide the nutrients he deems necessary to the plant directly to the root.
>
> The judgment that modern agriculture works effectively rests on a narrowly defined goal—that of maximized production. If we substitute goals of quality nutrition, general health and well being, or long-term survival of an agricultural system, the judgment of whether the system works might alter. There is no opportunity to judge the success of contemporary agriculture in terms of other goals, because contemporary science is not constituted to ask such questions, let alone try to answer them.[1]

The natural gardener will tell you that healthy soil means healthy plants, which means healthy animals and healthy people. Organic gardening appeals to the ecology-minded because it carries out the natural cycle designed for man to live by, the infinite details of which scientists are still, and perhaps forever, in the process of trying to determine.

The argument that manufacturers of chemical fertilizers wage against the organic gardener is that their own chemical processes fight against blight and insects and that their scientific agricultural techniques have made food more abundant and cheaper. The organic gardener maintains, however, that when natural methods are used, they do not have such hazards, and after a few years the soil is fertile enough to reduce fertilizing to a minimum. This is being done today on some large-scale commercial farms and thousands of smaller gardens. It is simply a matter of getting organized along the right lines. Many say that the continued use of manufactured fertilizers which lack certain important elements, such as trace minerals, will eventually lead to a sterile hardpan soil or dust bowl.

Beatrice Trum Hunter, author of an illuminating and instructive book *Gardening without Poisons,* points out that changes in gardening and farming practices will not be realized until an aroused public understands the issues. And the issues concern us all: the consumer of food as well as the tiller of soil. She claims that our practices are producing soils with lower vitality, plants with less vigor, less natural resistance, and reduced nutritive value. These unbalanced situations attract the pests which, in turn, grow more and more resistant as newer and stronger poisons are developed to try to conquer them, and our dilemma grows graver every year. Hunter contends that gardening without poisons in a backyard garden or in a large commercial operation is possible if we make use of the knowledge and tools we already possess. This I have witnessed for myself in our son's own large, pest-free, abundantly productive, organic garden.

Catharyn Elwood, another expert with splendid credentials, degrees, and life-long study in food and nutrition, explains organic gardening in her book *Feel Like A Million.* She first tells the horror story of the Food and Drug investigators who tested twenty-five meals gathered at different public eating places and found DDT residues in every food, which included meat, fried and mashed potatoes, pie, and coffee with cream.

They came to the conclusion that "few," if any, foods today can be found that are entirely free of DDT. The battle over DDT raged for a long time with pressure groups bearing down on its use. Finally new rulings were made to eliminate DDT.

Elwood explains that with present-day farming methods, only two inches of the original nine inches of topsoil have not been mined away. Furthermore, the farmer has used stimulating fertilizers to blow up what is left into false production of food. This assault, plus not returning natural produce to the soil—vegetable and animal wastes—has destroyed organic matter which actually *is* the life of the soil. This dark organic material, humus, offers nourishment which makes plants disease resistant so they can be grown without sprays. It is the deficient plant that becomes infested with pests. Elwood reasons that these pests appear by instinct for the purpose of returning some green matter into the soil in order to keep a living balance! In view of what we learn in organic gardening, we see again, as we see in degerminating grain, that man in turning to his own ways removes life—life with its life-giving properties.

Elwood quotes Louis Bromfield in a significant testimony before the House Select Committee in which he frankly stated his belief in organic gardening:

> The increasing attack by insects and disease upon agriculture and horticulture has risen largely through poor and greedy agricultural methods, through the steady deterioration of soils and the steady loss of organic materials . . . and the increasing unavailability of the natural elements through the loss and destruction of soil structures and content. In other words, a sick soil produces sick and weakened plants which are immediately subject to disease and insect attack. . . . I myself farmed and gardened in France for seventeen years on land that had been in use for twelve hundred years without ever using a dust or spray. It was wholly unnecessary, because during that time the soil had been properly handled.[2]

We can be relieved, at least, that recently two dangerous and most widely used pesticides have been forced off the market. They are aldrin and dieldrin (into which aldrin breaks down after it is used). The Environmental Protection Agency has ordered the Shell Chemical Company to stop manufacturing these two highly toxic chemicals which they say are an imminent hazard to our health. They accumulate in fatty tissues when taken into the body and are suspected of causing cancer on the basis of tests made on rats and mice.

The EPA cites tests showing that measurable amounts of dieldrin were found in 83% of all dairy products sampled and 96% of meat, fish, and poultry. More than 90% of the two pesticides produced in the country are in the soil in corn fields. Again we are faced with the fact that dangerous chemicals which can find their way into our bodies are allowed by the FDA and USDA to be used on a large scale until, and unless, forced off the market by other agencies. This gives further credence to Hunter's statement that gardening and farming practices will not be changed until an aroused public understands the issues. Is it not a part of Christian stewardship to investigate the issues which reliable researchers say threaten our health now and for generations to come? Ignorance may be costly.

Organic gardening does insure us of the natural elements we know to be necessary to health. But, as stated before, there are not only elements that science has not yet identified, but there are elements that are identified whose exact relationship to health is not known. Exciting discoveries are being made. An example concerns recent discoveries about trace elements. They are found to play a dramatic part in our physical and mental well-being. I go into more detail on this later but want to touch at this point upon their relationship to organic gardening. Robert Rodale tells us that we have allowed a system of agriculture to develop that cuts off the route by which trace element stores used to be recycled, and we have compounded the problem by eating more highly processed foods from which the great bulk of trace element stores are systematically removed.[3]

The preservation of trace elements is now definitely recognized as essential to good physical and mental health. And these trace elements, according to Frank A. Gilbert, author of *Mineral Nutrition and the Balance of Life,* are found in liberal amounts in organic material.[4] He also reminds us that all the trace elements we will ever have are here now—no more are being made. Consequently, we must be sure they are kept in the food chain to assure ourselves maximum health.

Robert Rodale says that trace elements generally being defined as those which are vital to human and animal, and even plant health, are present and effective in minute quantities. He is emphatic about the balance needed in trace elements because some have potential for harm if one is exposed to an excessive quantity. For that reason, Rodale recommends natural approaches to them. Certain natural foods, such as organ meats, bones, and whole grains, tend to accumulate trace elements. Whole grains are important trace element sources because the reproduction germ of a seed is another concentration point for these "tiny keys" to better health. Most important of all, Rodale admonishes, avoid white sugar which has the ability to drain trace element resources from other foods in an average diet.

Colin Fisher, Director of Britain's Pye Research Centre, has said, "With the price of fertilizer going up the way it is, it looks as if organic gardening will soon be the only way food can be grown economically at all." [5] However, neither our agricultural department nor agri-businesses are going to be convinced. The only way they see to meet the tragic and staggering problem of world food shortages, the field labor shortage, and various other economic and political problems is to continue on the course the nation has cut out for itself.

We are told that with improved fertilizers farmers will produce 40% more per acre than they do now. We do not hear about the nutritional value of the crops nor the subsequent quality of the soil—that remains to be seen. Feeding starving nations is, of course, an important world concern. But, when the experts discuss nutrition in this context, they simply mean food—any food. Even depleted food can save the starving from death. However, the only sensible, ultimate answer is to introduce higher nutritive value crops and better quality soil to these poor countries.

Our Department of Agriculture speaks only in terms of supplying manufactured chemical fertilizers to poor nations; counter to this, there is a constructive move toward organic gardening by the United Nations. An organic agricultural project is being developed in Nairobi in the form of an ecological farm. According to the U.N., "An ecological farm is a farm respecting the environment and trying to use as many inputs as possible, such as solar energy, wind energy, manure, and so forth. Such a farm, they say, aims at producing as many natural products as possible such as milk without DDT, fruit without pesticides, butter without artificial ingredients, etc." [6]

Many of us take heart that there may be a change of attitude about organic gardening in the United States when we read an article by Joan Dye Gassow, an instructor at Columbia University Teachers College Program in Nutrition, in which she says:

> As nutrition professionals, we have long been taught to view organic agriculture and the food it produces as one of the more extreme of the "fads" with which we must regularly contend. . . . Though many people in nutrition find it surprising, the fact is that a growing number of thoughtful people concerned with ecology, agriculture and the world food supply, support, or at least take seriously, the experiments being conducted by organic agriculturists.[7]

Whether or not the food dilemma is insurmountable, as agri-business believes it to be on any other farming basis than the one they have adopted, the fact remains that we are free as citizens, and Christians, to farm and to eat as our consciences dictate. Nature's pattern in gardening is rewarding privately or commercially.

Raising Animals

In regard to raising animals organically, there is much going on in agri-business these days which is a great departure from the laws of nature. It involves the grass animals graze on, the feed they consume, and the way they are raised, which includes the use of medication, pesticides, and insecticides.

Beatrice Trum Hunter compares the former way of raising beef cattle with our practices today. She reminds us how cattle valued as good beef with flavor matured slowly in the pasture and then went directly to slaughter. Now, only about twenty years later, the quality and nutritive value are largely ignored in an intense search for economy, speed, and bigness—a radical change. The fertility of the pasture may be undermined by repeated applications of synthetic fertilizers, drugs, and pesticides, all of which affect the livestock. Then the animals are fattened quickly and cheaply to get them to market sooner and sell them at maximum profit. Many of the practices, Hunter says, run counter to the health of the livestock and the safety of the food. She says that forcing practices can only be maintained by continuous use of antibiotics, vaccines, serums, and other medications, and as a result the basic physiology of the animal has been altered. Beef animals, twelve to eighteen months old, may be confined to feed lots and encouraged to overeat fattening foods. Drugs may be given that change the metabolism and increase fat artificially—fat which is hard, white, and almost totally saturated.[8] (Another reason, perhaps, that we are advised to eat lean meat—the fat is not really natural fat!)

Ross Hume Hall informs us that "as each new antibiotic was released for human medicine, it was also pressed into service as a growth promoter for livestock. . . . the FDA estimates that 78% of the meat and eggs consumed in the United States comes from animals fed medicated feeds." [9] He goes on to say that Dr. C. D. Van Houweling, Director of the Bureau of Veterinary Medicine of the FDA, emphasizes the value of antibiotics to livestock technology: They stimulate growth and enhance survival of cattle, swine, poultry, and other livestock. He quotes Van Houweling as saying, "Antibiotics are most effective in the early growing period and in warding off disease in animals that are crowded or improperly housed or malnourished." [10] This certainly leaves nothing to the imagination of the consumer. Such remarks from the FDA, if nothing else, put us on notice about the accepted farming conditions and methods in our country. "After twenty years of antibiotic use," Hall tells us, "agricultural scientists have failed to arrive at any understanding of what physiologic systems are affected or what biochemical transformations might be taking place in the flesh." [11]

Many of us followed the DES (diethylstibestrol, a synthetic growth hormone) battle for years. This hormone was fed to poultry as well as to cattle and sheep because it was a boon to business; animals grew faster and bigger on less feed at less expense. According to quite a detailed report in *Eating May Be Hazardous to Your Health,* the world's leading experts on cancer causation thought it should be banned.[12] Besides this, twenty-one countries, some as far back as 1959, had forbidden the use of growth-promoting hormones, including DES, as a cattle-fattening agent because of health dangers. And some countries deliberately banned the importation of our beef because of it. Canada was the most recent until the USDA promised that we would send them beef from animals which had not been fed DES. We remember the speeches Commissioner Charles Edwards of the FDA made to gain public support in which he praised industry and attacked the consumer advocates, Ralph Nader and Morton Mintz, saying that "the voice of responsible science must rise above the din. If not, the 'special interests,' the zealots, and the extremists will drown out the voice of reason" and said that "DES was a case in point." [13]

The FDA continued to allow DES, until finally in 1973, after eight years of congressional hearings, a consumer lawsuit, and threatened federal legislation, the FDA attempted to ban its use. But in January, 1974, the U.S. Court of Appeals overturned the ban because of "disputed facts." Representative Fountain, one of our congressmen who worked hard and long getting DES banned, said that it took all those years and all that pressure to get the FDA to perform its stated duty—to protect our food supply. After all that, in January, 1976, we are still not protected.

Dr. Alexander Schmidt, present commissioner of the FDA says:

> DES is still on the market because of a court's interpretation of the law. It is an admitted carcinogen, and we banned it in 1972 as an additive in animal feed because it left residues in the meat.
>
> But a court overturned us and said that before we can take such action, we had to have a hearing. Some of our hearings have gone on for two years. When the lawyers go to work, they often remove the action from the scientists— from the people who can best make benefit/risk decisions.
>
> We have again proposed a ban of DES as an animal-feed additive. If somebody wants a hearing, we'll hold one. We cannot ban it until this process is completed.[14]

It looks as though the "zealots" and the "extremists" will have to persevere.

The long and complicated story of DES, though briefly reviewed, is simply a warning to those of us who wish to be alerted to what is still going on in raising animals for human consumption. Verrett tells us that the DES case "was only a single limited victory in a much larger battle." She maintains that the focus of the DES controversy "could well have been any of about one hundred other drugs still given to animals through feed, many of them as potentially dangerous as DES." [15] For example, she says there are fourteen other synthetic hormones like DES in use in feed which many scientists believe to have the same cancer-producing properties as DES. The FDA itself has classified ten hormones as proven or potential carcinogens.

It is hard to believe we have become such a drug-oriented, profit-motivated country that we accept the practices of agribusiness and their reasoning without question. It would seem when we overlook quality and accept unnatural environment outwardly or inwardly for ourselves or our livestock, that we, as stewards of God's natural provisions for us, need to start questioning and investigating the situation before it is too late.

When it comes to antibiotics, Verrett tells us that about half the nation's entire antibiotic output, or $50,000,000 worth, goes directly into the feed for animals intended for human consumption to make them gain weight faster and keep them disease-free. In 1972 the FDA scientists listed the drugs which, if misused, can leave illegal residues in animal tissue. They listed thirty-three in cattle, forty-seven in poultry, twenty-seven in swine, fourteen in sheep, twenty-six in milk, eighteen in eggs, and even two in fish. The significant point is that it is possible for these drugs to get into animal tissue, milk, and eggs and that scientists claim that in nearly all cases the controls (mainly the withdrawal times of the drugs in feed before slaughter) were inadequate to prevent residues and assure the safety of food. This was the case with DES.

Medical experts say there is no way to ascertain what affect various residues of antibiotics will have on different people, but they do say that they pose problems. One problem is the building up of resistance to antibiotics, rendering them useless when needed. (Antibiotic ointments for cuts and scratches were taken off the over-the-counter market for this reason.) Another problem is that the USDA admits to not having good techniques available to detect residues in tissue.

We do have an Antibiotic Task Force set up by the FDA after a British scientist's report urging an end to the use of antibiotics in animal feed. Our task force urged stern restrictions on drugs in animal feed, but, Verrett says, a year later the FDA had taken no action. There is another "disheartening situation," Verrett reports, and that is the government's permitting a number of drugs in medicated feed which it never then checks for residues. There is a law, she says, which requires producers to provide a practicable method for detecting residues, but it is not enforced. "As long as the FDA and the USDA continue to systemically violate the law, a string of potentially dangerous drugs will continue to plague us as unknown hazards."[16] This is a sobering statement coming from a researcher with fifteen years' experience with the FDA.

The same unnatural farming methods are used in raising poultry. Poultry raisers use medicated feed; the farmer is trusted to read all labels and abide strictly by instructions to discontinue use at a specified point before slaughter, but we have many reports of birds reaching the market contaminated with illegal excessive residues of medicine. The point in question for the consumer is: as long as medicated feed is allowed at all, how do we know about the chicken we buy at the market?

In Europe the consumer does not have to ask that question; they don't allow medicated feed, and American poultry is being subjected to severe restrictions in many European countries. It is considered substandard under certain European food health laws, Hunter informs us in her report entitled "Europe Turns Thumbs Down." "For example, in 1965 the French Ministry of Health banned the use of all antibiotics, hormones, and other drugs in the feed of animals intended for human consumption. The importation of poultry raised on additives of doubtful safety, such as arsenicals, and others, is prohibited."[17] The USDA doesn't like this and tries to get rules changed abroad. We hope instead that the World Codex Alimentarius will force some changes in American husbandry. We do know that we were the only nation out of forty to give a dissenting vote at the World Health Organization of the U.N. for "wider consideration of the technological efficacy and justification for the use of food additives, especially food standards issued by the Codex Alimentarius Commission."

Buying Meat and Poultry

Marketing for meat and poultry presents a problem if you do not have access to produce from organic farms, which is the case with most of us. As we are told in the *Supermarket Handbook*, "Beef is the most available, most popular, and the most tainted. This is the meat that most often boasts a USDA grading shield."[18]

At the time of writing this book, the export-import meat situation is under debate because of our depressed market. I am interested in boosting our own economy, but must admit that I would get beef from Canada and lamb from New Zealand, or any meat from anywhere if it is meat which has not been subjected to drugs and growth hormones. If we are fortunate enough to be able to purchase organically grown meat (meat from animals which have grazed on pastures which are not fertilized with manufactured chemicals or sprayed with pesticides and animals which are not fed drugs and growth-promoting hormones), it is the safest. Otherwise, it is wise to know your butcher and the condition of his shop—many are not sanitary. The most nutritious meat is organ meat—liver, heart, kidneys, and such. Veal is safer than beef because young animals do not go through the final fattening-up process with medicated feed.

The cut of beef we must be most careful about is ground beef. In grinding the meat, the tissues are broken down and the fluids released are a perfect culture for bacteria. Have your beef ground fresh and use it up in a day or two. Otherwise, wrap it well and freeze it.

Avoid hot dogs, luncheon meats, and most sausage. Reading the labels is enough to make you pass them by, but the label does not begin to tell you the full story: meat packers don't have to throw away what they trim off of meat for retail purposes because they can sell the trimmings to us along with other animals parts they could not sell if identified, such as cheeks, lips, jowls, heads, and veal carcasses. We eat them with their high fat content (30 to 50%), their sugar, and their assortment of chemicals. We do this to the tune of 2,000,000,000 pounds a year according to *Consumers Research* magazine.[19] Needless to say, these meats are very profitable to the meat packer but hardly beneficial to the consumer. Avoid them. Slice your own meat for lunches and picnics.

According to the illustration on the jacket of Dr. Jacobson's book *Eater's Digest,* the actual content of a hot dog is 28% fat, 56% water, and 40% carbohydrate fillers with the additives we should avoid: sodium nitrate, sodium erythorbate, and artificial coloring. The carbohydrate fillers include corn syrup and dextrose. In this unenticing combination we come out with only 12% protein for the entire hot dog which weighs one ounce. The protein value some of us counted upon in frankfurters is so little that it figures out to cost fifteen dollars a pound. And this, with a thick bun made of depleted flour, is what we lovingly put into our children's dear little bodies!

John McClure warns us vividly in his book *Meat Eaters Are Threatened* that we are safest buying our meat right from the wholesaler and butchering it ourselves.[20] This requires knowing a reliable butcher and having a large deep freeze or frozen food locker, but it is also economical. If you can buy organically grown meat a side at a time, you are making a sound investment in both product safety and nutritive value.

If possible, purchase turkey direct from the farm instead of frozen in the supermarket. In the November, 1973, *Consumer Reports* Jim Hightower dispelled any illusion we might have about the little processing frozen turkey must undergo. Are turkeys simply cleaned well, wrapped, and frozen? Not so, he says: "The major sellers of frozen turkey add fat, sodium, sugar, artificial color, and artificial flavor, not to mention emulsifiers, flavor enhancers, antioxidants, and other chemicals."[21] Hightower also explained the addition of water in the processing of turkeys. He said that it is legal for processors to add sodium phosphate to turkey, which causes it to hold water. Quoting *Consumer Reports,* he further explained "a peculiar chain of circumstances" that occurs at the turkey factory:

> A turkey (1) will absorb water during processing. Therefore (2) processors gain permission to sell turkey with water added. But (3) the absorbed water seeps out. So (4) the processors use chemicals to retain at least as much water as they're allowed to add. Then they (5) sell water at turkey prices, implying that (6) water makes turkey taste better.[22]

Now we know what some of us are paying for and eating on Thanksgiving!

Perhaps we would like to know a little more about our Easter ham, too. We do know that hams do not taste the same as they used to and certainly do not have the same good texture. Hams are now "the bland, chemically processed, water-filled, plastic-wrapped simulations of modern industry."[23] And, as we know, ham is cured with sodium nitrite. Hightower describes the evolution of ham thus: "Big business moved into the ham industry, expanding well beyond the scale that makes quality control possible, and they were far too eager for profits to wait for the slow-curing process that decent ham flavor requires. Why wait when a heavy dose of chemicals and a heavier dose of advertising will produce bigger profits than quality?"[24]

Government Standards

Government standards in food are something else we would do well to understand. The standard arrived at is not necessarily fact or truth; it can be what producers are turning out economically with government sanctions. For example, the government has made standards for milk which are based on pasteurization. Therefore, any product from natural, whole, raw milk has to be labeled imitation! Another example of imposing false definitions on the public is in labeling spaghetti. The government decided that spaghetti is made from wheat flour, so any other spaghetti is not truly spaghetti. DeBoles spaghetti, for instance, which is made of Jerusalem artichoke flour and is delightfully suitable to those on low carbohydrate diets, must be labeled "imitation," when there is nothing imitation in it or about it.

There seems to be another side to the government's coin concerning imitation. "Dan Greenberg describes a recent FDA ruling that all but eliminates the requirement that *imitation* (my emphasis) foods be labeled imitation,"[25] writes Ross Hume Hall. As long as nutritional equivalents exist (a definition of nutritional which excludes many factors), the government thinks this is perfectly fair. The FDA defends this new ruling by contending that "it is made in the public interest, since to call a chemically fabricated product a chemically fabricated product would constitute 'a trade barrier against the introduction of nutritious new products.' "[26] Hall concludes: "This new regulation, and more importantly the attitude that lies behind it, plus the new regulations for nutritional labeling of foods, insure that the public will be completely cut off from organic forces.... the individual has now been placed completely at the disposal of the food fabricators."[27] If our generation does not demand honesty in labeling, the next generation never will know what true food is. When "imitation" stands for the real thing, and the imitated is not so identified, we see that action in getting industry and government back on the track is long overdue.

Furthermore, we must understand that government promotes and sanctions agricultural practices which produce vegetables and fruits with less nutritive value than natural produce and which are deceiving in their appearance. One of the ills is in mass production: for instance, the development of tomatoes. We are now learning that the Department of Agriculture spends millions of the taxpayers' money tailoring tomatoes to machines for mass production. Tomatoes must be developed which have thick, tough walls to withstand the abuse of being harvested by machinery. Thus, they are almost tasteless. Dr. Jean Mayer says:

> For too long, the nutritional value of fruits and vegetables has been overlooked and neglected in this country. Unfortunately, the qualities selected in the breeding of "improved" varieties have been entirely related to external appearances and to the convenience of harvesters, shippers, and processors. What is more, the harvesting and "ripening" practices show little regard for preserving the nutritional contents, particularly in respect to vitamins and minerals.... The tomato, 1973 style, is a whole new thing. Millions of dollars worth of research have been successfully applied to produce what California nutritionist Audrey T. Cross has called "a clockwork tomato." In its perfection, it is hard, not juicy; uniform in size and shape, not plump; and above all, it has to be tough enough to be picked by automatic harvesters, tumbled through a mechanized assembly line, and shipped thousands of miles—all without telltale bruises.

As for the nutritional content, one tomato recently developed at Purdue University is being heralded as potentially a great commercial success because of its uniform shape— yet, when ripe, it will at best contain approximately half the vitamin A content of the varieties of tomatoes presently on the market. But wait, there is worse to come. Most tomatoes we are eating now are not vine ripened but are being picked green in Southern climates and artificially "ripened" by spraying them with ethylene gas in special chambers! Both from the viewpoint of taste and that of nutrition, such a tomato is inferior to one that is ripened on the vine.[28]

One wonders if the day will come when the beautiful, tender nutritious, garden-grown, hand-picked tomato will be called "imitation" because it is not grown by the standards devised for mass production. We know that ethlyene gas is used to turn green fruit the color of ripened fruit (oranges are probably the best-known example); so, with all the protection the government is supposed to be giving us, we have no idea about some things we are buying. Mayer tells us that ethylene gas can turn a green tomato red and make it look ripe; hence, since green tomatoes can be in any stage of ripening, the practice of picking them and reddening them means there is a good chance that we will buy unripe fruit. *Consumers Report,* January, 1974, issue, cites a random survey conducted by scientists in Florida who found in one shipment of so-called "mature" green Florida tomatoes that 40% were not ripe. In another shipment, 78% were not ripe.

There seems to be no end to the measures taken by industry, with the government's sanction, which confuse the public and subordinate the natural and the more nutritious. And we wonder what is causing some of our stomach aches!

We can ask ourselves whether this is the way our country is supposed to operate? Our government was founded as a nation under God, governed by the people and for the people. We, the people, are the sovereignty, not agri-business, not appointed bureaucrats, not even elected officials—hence the Constitution clearly sets forth the channels by which the people can change abuses. Isn't it ironic that countries under other forms of government have shown more concern and protection for their people in the food they consume than our country has? The profiteers in foreign food industry apparently are not the decision-makers. We, the people, when we know something to be wrong, should go through all proper channels to change it.

Furthermore, as Christians, we all feel strongly about not contributing to the furtherance of wrong standards. We also feel strongly about not tolerating anything corrupt or impure in any area of life. Pollution is corruption in a very real sense— corruption of the body. Food pollution is one of the pollutions we can each do something about today, both by what we eat and by what stand we take. Second Corinthians 7:1 says: "Let us turn away from everything wrong, whether of body or of spirit" (LIVING BIBLE).

Convenience Foods

A number of the processed foods we need to avoid have been briefly described. But we also have to consider the growing assortment of convenience foods. Most have undergone several of the aforementioned processes and contain some, often many, additives. On top of this, many will be cooked for the second time in our kitchens. Besides the fact that they are, for the most part, poor in flavor and usually inferior in quality, they are expensive. Avoid canned and frozen meat products when looking for food value and monetary value. We are getting very little meat and are paying a lot of money for a lot of additives, extenders, and packaging. In canned meat, we are told, we are getting the cheapest, most undesirable parts of animals doctored up with spices and chemicals. Read the labels, and you will find the usual offenders—nitrates and nitrites, MSG, hydrolyzed plant protein, and sugar, among others. To enlighten you about the percentages of meat found in meat products, here are a few frozen products as shown in the *Supermarket Handbook.*

> Veal Parmigiana—40% breaded meat
> Meat Pies—25% meat
> Lasagne—12% meat
> Entrees of meat, gravy, and one vegetable—30% meat
> Meat Casseroles—25% uncooked meat or 18% cooked[29]

Just as we need no longer live under the illusion that we are serving good quality protein and acceptable meals when we serve hot dogs, luncheon meats, and most sausages, we need not live under the illusion that canned and frozen meat products and other convenience foods compare nutritionally or economically with homemade foods. The most economical and nutritious way to eat today is to make things ourselves from natural, fresh foods properly cooked without chemical additives.

In the first part of my book I spoke briefly on the subject of our pace of living. I would like to mention it again in relation to convenience foods. Where convenience foods are a way of life in a family, they not only provide less nutrition, but they contribute to the hurried pace of life in the home. They all too often do away with the leisurely enjoyment and fellowship of mealtime. Convenience foods can be served quickly, eaten quickly—even be eaten on the run. In fact, our television advertisements show this as an "asset"—the meal you can throw in as you are going out the door. This kind of eating does not bring relaxation, which we all need, and it is certainly hard on the digestion. Convenience foods keep us from making mealtime the special and joyful occasion it should be.

We do the most we can for ourselves and our families when we take time to carefully prepare meals from natural, unadulterated, untampered-with, God-given foods and take time to relish them together with a prayer of gratitude.

I am grateful for the stand so many youths are taking today in insisting upon eating only that which is natural. And they are taking time to cook it properly and eat it leisurely. I am grateful for the men in legislature who are taking an honest look at what cattle are being fed in feed lots where they are fattened. We can hope that the day will come when there will be so much public support that we will not have to serve Meat a la Antibiotic and a la Hormone for dinner. I am grateful for the number of health food stores which are mushrooming around the country.

I am grateful for the positive signs of organic gardening, and I am grateful for farms where animals are raised on feed which is properly fertilized on purer water and where they do not administer medicine for weight gain. I am grateful for the people who are taking enough interest in fertilizers and pesticides to voice their opinions in Washington. And I am grateful for the men and women in Washington who are doing their utmost—with little, if any, support from most of us—to eliminate the present hazards in foods. With the health of the nation at stake, we should all be supporting them. How strange it is that most of our nation's leaders will take a stand on air and water pollution but not on food pollution which affects the nation's bodies, minds, and nervous systems; to the contrary, they endorse the refined, the highly processed, the imitation, the additives, and the foodless foods.

Lastly, I have been grateful and indebted all my life to the men and women in the field of nutrition who have withstood the irresponsible attacks from so many quarters—segments of medicine, industry, and bureaucracy—and have continued to forge ahead with their research on food for the sake of mankind. Profit has not been the motive; they have taken the hard road. Going against the tide is the hardest way to earn a living, and it is both physically and emotionally draining. I believe the time has come when evidence is sufficient for men and women of conscience to back them. We can most effectively do this by marketing wisely, eating well, reading on the subject, keeping up with legislation, and being willing to write our congressmen and women.

PART 3

Preventive Medicine

Do you want to get well?

John 5:6

Chapter 7

Preventive Medicine Versus

Crisis Medicine

In the King James Version of the Bible the word "whole" is used to mean physical health. Jesus continually used the word "whole." He told the woman with the issue of blood that her faith had made her "whole" (Luke 8:48); He told Jairus that his daughter was made "whole" (Matt. 15:28); all the diseased of Gennesaret were made "perfectly whole" (Matt. 14:36); the centurion's servant was found "whole that had been sick" (Luke 7:10); and the man with the withered hand had it restored "whole as the other" (Luke 6:10).

Later translations use various words to replace "whole," such as "healed," "well," and "restored." Whatever the translation, the idea of wholeness and completeness is implied. We are intended to be whole; when we are whole, we are completely well. Wholeness physically, then, must mean the health of every cell of the body—a condition in which disease cannot start. This is the condition with which preventive medicine concerns itself.

The tragic fact in society today is that preventive medicine and traditional medicine are two different fields. They should work together; all too often they work apart. The reason that these two fields rarely come together is that medical education is on its own drug-oriented track. The majority of medical schools do not teach nutrition. Likewise, the American Medical Association is preoccupied with drugs and does not recognize the importance of nutrition. Although less than half of the physicians in the country belong to the AMA, its views are still considered authoritative by many. Dr. Russell Roth, president of the AMA, says: "Medicine's job is to educate and encourage people to give early attention to disease." Preventive medicine's job, on the other hand, is to maintain a condition in which disease does not take hold. Dr. Roger Williams says:

> The most basic weapons in the fight against disease are those most ignored by modern medicine: *the numerous nutrients that the cells of our bodies need.* If our body cells are ailing—as they must in disease—the chances are excellent that it is because they are being inadequately provisioned. The list of the things that these cells may need includes not only all the amino acids and all the minerals, plus trace elements, but about fifteen vitamins and probably many other coenzymes, nutrilites, and metabolites.[1]

Williams goes on to observe that physicians, with their background and knowledge as to how our bodies are built and how they function, are precisely the ones who should qualify to develop expertise in this area. To date, the majority do not. Their approach is to try to find out what is wrong with a patient by giving whichever of today's four thousand available tests they choose. If these tests identify something, the doctors prescribe the appropriate medicine and treatment if they can. They do not go into the nutritional aspect of health; what one eats has no place on their medical history forms, and they usually do not discuss with us what we eat in any detail.

It stands to reason that if our bodies function best by consuming nutrients designed by nature for our health, a deficiency of these nutrients would cause certain disorders and disease both physically and mentally. It would also follow that the way to correct such disorders and disease would be the replacement of the nutrients—the vitamins, minerals, and other elements—which are lacking. This is the first premise of preventive medicine: we should eat what we need as well as avoid that which is harmful or unnecessary. Secondly, we should correct insufficiencies before a crisis occurs which demands drugs or surgery. Thirdly, at the crisis stage—the illness stage—the nutrients should be administered along with whatever other medical measures are determined necessary.

Medicine as it is practiced today has been described as "crisis medicine." Crisis medicine does not treat the patient for his ailment until symptoms have developed. The symptoms are the crisis which bring medical action.

The day of recognizing the intrinsic import of preventive medicine is at hand. In fact, it must be recognized if we are to survive. Lives are being saved by antibiotics as well as the other wonders of medicine; dreaded epidemics are being wiped out by inoculation; but all our degenerative and chronic ills continue to mount at an appalling rate.

The strides being made today in preventive medicine are more than encouraging—they are exciting. Doctors by the hundreds are becoming more aware of the necessity for the new approach to medicine. This is demonstrated by the thousands of doctors who wrote to Washington opposing the FDA regulations concerning vitamins. It is also demonstrated by the growing membership of preventive medical and nutritional societies. Furthermore, a large portion of our nation as a whole, thanks to the undaunted efforts of the specialists in the field, are becoming aware of the fact that there is a positive course to take to reduce physical, dental, and mental problems in our country.

As I see it, the positive course of preventive medicine covers several areas. First, it concerns itself with our daily nutrition and our general health beginning in the cradle. Second, it has to do specifically with the relationship between what we eat and how it affects the brain from the prenatal stage through life. Out of the tremendous research in these areas has emerged a new field of preventive medicine known as orthomolecular disease, including orthomolecular psychiatry. Another related field covers allergic and environmental diseases which stem from the chemicals in our food and in our present environmental conditions.

Chapter 8

The Role Daily Nutrition Plays in

Preventive Medicine

Dr. Emanuel Cheraskin,[1] one of our most knowledgeable exponents of preventive medicine, has pointed out that in China people pay doctors to keep them well. If this were the case in our country, a doctor would be forced to study nutrition or lose his practice. The nation is not staying well on the present basis of treating a person only when his disorder or disease has gone far enough to be named and attacked with a drug or a knife.

To discover the deficiencies and imbalances which lead to disorders and diseases is the objective of preventive medicine. The procedure entails a knowledge of nutrition and biochemistry beyond that possessed by most doctors. There is hope that in the future doctors will study nutrition in medical school and employ the expertise of nutritional biochemists (not just dieticians) in their practice, or refer their patients to people with competence in this area. This would enable doctors to provide for us the specific instruction in nutrition which is so vital to our health.

In this country, growing old is accompanied by many

disorders. Doctors would have us accept them as inevitable. Nutritional experts, however, are certain that they are *not* inevitable. They see these disorders as stemming from deficiencies, many of which can be treated.

There is also the obligation of a doctor to learn about what one can do *early* in life to help avoid the chronic ills of old age. I remember when I was in my teens telling my doctor, an eminent man in his field, that my mother had had arthritis and asking him what I could do to avoid it in my old age. The answer was that there was nothing I could do. I have since learned that people with either osteoarthritis or rheumatoid arthritis show marked deficiencies in certain minerals and vitamins, and I have learned that the proper administration of these elements, along with a nutritious diet, can make a startling difference to a large number of arthritics, young and old.

It would seem that if doctors, instead of accepting what they call inevitable, checked out any deficiencies in our youth and prescribed for them then, untold misery in later years could be lessened if not completely avoided. Eating nutritiously is mandatory, but being checked out for possible existing deficiencies due to heredity, environment, and other factors is also essential in preventing illness in later years.

As it is, many millions suffer and die of degenerative diseases. Cancer is one of them. Arthritis is another. There are 13,000,000 arthritics in our country. Many of these are in extreme pain, are unable to hold jobs, and many are bedridden. They live on aspirin. In severe cases they must be given stronger pain killers and sedatives. And they live on an atrocious diet. A few turn, as a last resort, to nutrition. The long-suffering arthritic, however, has all too often reached the point of eating almost nothing. Furthermore, he has set likes, dislikes, and habits he has no intention of changing. Added to this, he may have no teeth, like millions of others in our "healthy" country, and may have to wear dentures which really do not work well and limit his chewing capabilities. Also, he cannot believe that substantial amounts of vitamins and minerals will do him any good because he has heard the doctors downgrade their value (even though these doctors have not substantially helped his arthritis). And arthritis is only one of the many degenerative diseases which plague our nation.

Dr. Cheraskin, who spoke on predictive, or anticipatory, medicine at the March, 1973, conference of the International Academy of Preventive Medicine, gave an interesting account of what he terms the pluses and minuses for good health. He did his research on a group of physicians who cooperated with him, and following are some of his findings: the doctors with fewest complaints were those whose protein intake was high, who ate unrefined carbohydrates, who ate a greater amount of fats than the others, and who took vitamin and mineral supplements. Those with the highest number of complaints ate refined carbohydrates (starches and sugar). It was as simple as that. Yet, few people make a distinction between refined and unrefined carbohydrates, many overdo polyunsaturates and exclude saturated fats from their diets, the majority are not aware of what foods contain the best quality protein, and many have little understanding of supplementation.

Most people do not correlate what they eat with their complaints or their ability to resist disease. Cheraskin's theory is that the body makes sense, and that what is good for one part of the body is good for the whole body. This is certainly borne out in his findings that the doctors who ate wisely had fewer complaints and higher resistance to disease.

When are we going to start identifying the pluses and the minuses in our diets? When are we going to seriously examine our own daily nutrition?

Chapter 9

Prenatal Nutrition in Preventive Medicine

In his book *Nutrition Against Disease,* Dr. Roger J. Williams asserts that "If all prospective human mothers could be fed as expertly as prospective animal mothers in the laboratory, most sterility, spontaneous abortions, stillbirths, and premature births would disappear; the birth of deformed and mentally retarded babies would be largely a thing of the past." [1] He also says that mental development during infancy is fostered only if the nutrition is good. Williams is one of our distinguished scientists; he served for twenty years as Director of the Clayton Biochemical Institute. His statements bring great hope for more abundant health, physically and mentally, for future generations.

Dr. Philip Roos, executive director of the National Association for Retarded Children, spoke at the Southwest Regional Conference of the Association in June, 1973. During an interview following his speech he said that we must still emphasize the obvious in preventing retardation in babies: good diet and good prenatal care will help prevent mental retardation. Dr. Montgomery C. Hart, in a lecture on "The Neonatologist's View

97

of Nutrition," spoke of the fact that malnutrition of the fetus affects the brain. Mental retardation, he claims, is almost always due to malnutrition which can cause the loss of 60% of the brain cells.

Inasmuch as there are 6,000,000 mentally retarded individuals in our country, the added dimension of educating the public to the importance of prenatal nutrition would seem paramount. I have quoted only a few of the individuals concerned with prenatal care; there are many specialists in the field, and there is a great deal of technical information available on the relationship between the development of the brain and proper prenatal nutrition.

This, then, is the message: civilized, twentieth-century men and women have to go back and relearn what primitive man did by instinct. We must eat real food with special attention to prenatal nourishment.

Chapter 10

Orthomolecular Medicine and Psychiatry

A significant new field is developing which is related to preventive medicine. It is known as "orthomolecular medicine." The men and women who lead this dynamic field represent all branches of medicine, biochemistry, and nutrition. The orthomolecular theory holds that disease is most effectively treated through the restoration of normal elements to the body. This means bringing the chemistry of the bodily system into balance. "Ortho" means "right" (or correct); hence, the new term designates the right molecule in the right amount.

Orthomolecular is distinct from molecular medicine in that substances that are foreign to the body are not used in orthomolecular medicine; this is not the case in most molecular medicine. The idea is that there is some optimal level for each of the human substances that is consistent with complete health. Scientists have various ways of determining the optimal levels. One test that is being used today is the hair test. This method entails simply clipping strands of hair from the nape of the neck and from them making an analysis of the mineral content of the body. Dr. John Miller, former editor-in-chief of *Chemical Abstracts* and past president of the National Honorary Chemical Society, claims the hair test is the best diagnostic tool that has ever been found outside the biopsy (analysis of living body tissue).

A great deal of substantial work is coming out of the field of orthomolecular medicine including the treatment of mental disorders, or orthomolecular psychiatry. The day may be near when most of the mental and emotional disorders may be curable. We are told that one out of three families has a problem of serious mental illness, and the Association of Mental Health states that industry alone estimates that 85% of its accidents are due to mental and emotional problems.

Dr. Linus Pauling, who coined the word "orthomolecular," has contributed greatly to the field of mental health. Of particular interest to the medical profession is a book he edited with Dr. David Hawkins entitled *Orthomolecular Psychiatry.* There are also a number of other scientists and doctors who have done outstanding work in the field. Dr. Abram Hoffer of Canada is one. Hoffer, former Director of Psychiatric Research at the University of Saskatoon, Saskatchewan, has treated, among other types of mental problems, 2,500 cases of schizophrenia. His results have been extraordinary. He has reported a 93% cure for patients with combined therapy less than two years (not chronic). Hoffer explains, in his book *How to Live With Schizophrenia,* that schizophrenics need unusually large amounts of certain vitamins. Therefore, megavitamin therapy is necessary for effective treatment. There are various reasons why schizophrenics require large amounts of particular vitamins: one is that they have a vitamin deficiency; another is that they absorb only a part of the vitamins they ingest.

When we are told that "schizophrenia and depression, the two most prevalent mental disorders, affect more than 10 million Americans each year" [1] and the number increases in leaps and bounds, we know that traditional psychotherapy alone is not enough. "Previously the disorder (schizophrenia) had been wholly blamed on personal stresses, lack of adaptability or failure of the parents. Today, the biochemical basis is well documented." [2]

It is intriguing to think that Sigmund Freud characterized schizophrenia as chemical in origin and predicted a chemical cure. Now his original premise is being realized. One proof that "mental illness has a biochemical basis can be seen in the fact that symptoms can be switched off and on at will by adding or withdrawing megavitamin therapy—even when the patient is not aware of the change in treatment." [3] In order to test the theory of a chemical disturbance being responsible for schizophrenia, a psychiatrist injected himself with a concentration from the blood of schizophrenics called the MO factor. He was schizophrenic for two weeks until it worked out of him. It has also been discovered that if you inject a spider with a schizophrenic's blood, the spider will spin a distorted web. Dr. Carlton Fredericks, who tells of these experiments, also relates a supporting incident: twins were brought up separately and differently because they were adopted by different parents; at the age of twenty-two years and two months they each developed schizophrenia.

There is a Schizophrenics Anonymous patterned after Alcoholics Anonymous which is helping hundreds of people. SA uses the twelve traditions of AA, including the declaration of one's need for God. The major difference in them is the substitution of the word "schizophrenia" for "alcoholism."

Dr. Roger Williams sums it up when he says, "Even with our present state of knowledge, it should be possible both to prevent and to treat mental disease by attempting to furnish the patients everything needed for good brain nutrition."

Dr. Carl Pfeiffer is one of the doctors who has not neglected the biochemical aspects of mental illness and who is successfully treating this kind of illness. Pfeiffer is director of the Medical and Dental Staff of the New Jersey Neuropsychiatric Institute. He spoke at the 1973 seminar of the International Academy of Preventive Medicine, and in presenting his topic, "Trace Metal Treatment of Schizophrenia," he emphasized the important role of trace minerals, one of which is zinc. He explained that many people have an insufficient intake of zinc and that it is not well stored in the body; this can cause, or contribute to, problems, including psychological problems. For example, schizophrenics have about half the necessary amount of zinc.

Physical and mental disorders can, therefore, be caused by chemical imbalance. This imbalance, in turn, can be caused by deficiencies in particular vitamins, minerals, and other elements, or by an unusual need for them.

Mental and physical disorders can also be caused by allergy. This includes allergic and allergic-like susceptibilities as well as addictive responses to the toxic chemicals in our environment. Dr. Marshall Mandell, director of the New England Foundation of Allergic and Environmental Disease, says that man has gone millions of years without the symptoms we now have had for the past fifty years. He says our systems were not intended to cope with our present environment and all it entails. He maintains that a thorough knowledge of food allergy and chemical susceptibility is absolutely essential for all physicians in every branch of medicine. A significant portion of each medical practice consists of unrecognized allergic and addictive responses to environmental conditions that must be recognized if these disorders are to be treated correctly.

Dr. William Philpot, a psychiatrist and Associate Director of Fuller Memorial Sanitarium in South Attleboro, Massachusetts, goes so far as to say that all psychoses are organic in origin (a reaction to a chemical or a food), and that one-third of all neuroses fall into the same category. Dr. Philpot uses the word "maladaptive reactions" in describing the problems caused by certain foods and particular characteristics of our environment.

In summary, orthomolecular psychiatry provides a new and promising method of treating mental illness. Its guiding principle is that the functioning of the mind is dependent on the nutritional and chemical state of the brain.

Chapter 11

Preventive Medicine and Crisis Medicine—Will They Be Integrated?

Preventive medicine means wholeness. It means attaining and maintaining a physical condition in which disease does not start. It means paying attention to realistic prenatal preparation and building young bodies through proper nutrition to avoid as many later ills as possible. It means taking the necessary measures to reverse the present trend of our degenerative diseases. It means approaching physical and mental disease from a standpoint of possible chemical imbalances. It means being aware of the mental and physical effects of our present-day environment, including pollution of air, water, and food.

Fundamentally, preventive medicine means looking for the natural balance God intended for our bodies. It means achieving this balance to the greatest degree possible with substances natural to our bodies, intended for our bodies, compatible with our bodies. Preventive medicine means utilizing the significant findings of distinguished scientists, findings which come out of fifty years of thorough and continuing research.

Crisis medicine, on the other hand, means diagnosing

symptoms and alleviating or curing disease through drugs and sophisticated techniques. It means conquering infections and combating viruses with antibiotics. It means almost abolishing dreaded epidemics through immunization. It means setting bones, removing disabled organs, and grafting flesh. In fact, the achievements of crisis medicines are too many to enumerate.

The FDA, which is made up of medical traditionalists grounded in crisis medicine, has the important role of controlling the accuracy of labeling and of preventing the marketing and distribution of contaminated food and dangerous drugs.

Both preventive medicine and crisis medicine have important roles. Each is valuable and each needs the support, the insights, and the techniques of the other. Yet the benefits of their cooperation are not realized because of the antagonism of the medical traditionalists practicing crisis medicine towards those in the field of preventive medicine. For example, too often some of the members of the FDA and the AMA (which represents the medical traditionalists) dismiss all findings outside their own jurisdiction, especially those of preventive medicine, alleging that they are "premature," "uncontrolled," "irresponsible," and "unscientific."

The seeming reluctance of some of the medical traditionalists to accept research and discoveries from other sources is not new. For example, Louis Pasteur's germ theory, upon which much of medicine is hinged today, took many, many years to be accepted. And it took ten years and the pressures of World War II before traditional medicine would accept Dr. Alexander Fleming's discovery of penicillin. Surely the day will also come when medical traditionalists will accept the nutritional and orthomolecular approach as integral to their practice and essential to wholeness and health.

We may take heart: the number of competent doctors who are turning their attention to preventive medicine is increasing. There are many hundreds, and the number is growing. As for the number of orthomolecular psychiatrists: there were only a dozen a few years ago, and today they number in the hundreds. These physicians are concerned not only with our daily nutritional needs, but also with mental and emotional illnesses including alcoholism, drug abuse, senility, infant psychoses, autism, depression, and schizophrenia.

Chapter 12

Do We Have a Responsibility in

Preventive Medicine?

There is a constructive role we, the public, can play in the advancement of preventive medicine. We need to learn more about nutrition ourselves and practice it, and we need to voice informed opinions in Washington. Our government has done a good job in supporting crisis medicine; it has done nothing to support preventive medicine. If we are to survive, we must see that funds are channeled into *both* fields. The funds are badly needed. The experts in the overlapping fields of nutrition, biochemistry, and environmental and orthomolecular disease tell us that, despite their significant findings, they have just scratched the surface—a great deal of critical research has yet to be done.

There is also a constructive role for Christians to play in preventive medicine. We can develop new attitudes and take new, more effective action in our homes, our churches, and our communities. As Christians, we know we have a responsibility to understand and respect all the things of which we are stewards (among them, the fruits of the earth: grain, meat, eggs, vegetables—in other words, our food).

As Christians, we also share a responsibility to understand the needs of those to whom we are stewards (ourselves, our families, our fellow Christians, and others whom God would have us serve) and to put these needs in a specifically Christian context.

We need to see ourselves as whole persons, having bodies, minds, and spirits. God is a creator of integrated wholes, not separated fragments. It follows, therefore, that the biochemical balance He designs for our bodies influences our health—mental, physical, and emotional—and we have a responsibility to keep that balance.

As stewards to our young children we are, of course, responsible for their physical, spiritual, educational, and social needs. In addition, however, we are responsible for their emotional and psychological balance. If we are to meet their needs for balance, we must understand that there is a relationship between that balance and the food we provide for them. There is also a relationship between their patterns of behavior and the food they consume. (Later adolescent behavior that is unethical and antisocial may have nothing to do with lack of obedience or faith.) Preventive medicine can enable us to understand that there are these relationships, and it can suggest how we should provide accordingly. It can suggest, for example, how we should begin at the very beginning by providing proper prenatal nutrition. Furthermore, preventive medicine makes us aware of the kind of professional help we need for our children.

As stewards to our fellow Christians and to others, with the perspectives of preventive medicine, we can realize more quickly and more accurately what some of their urgent needs are. And we can act more directly and effectively in helping them meet those needs. For example, as lay persons, and particularly as pastors and counselors, we can realize that the problems brought to us may not be psychological or spiritual in origin but may be due to faulty diet and chemical imbalance. Having realized this, we can then suggest ways of dealing directly with the causes, or, if the problems are beyond our competence, we can recommend someone specializing in the area.

Every pastor, counselor, and lay person is faced with a challenge: can we develop new insights and attitudes toward mental and emotional problems, and will we initiate new action to cope with these problems? If we will, the future is promising indeed.

PART 4

Why We Eat the Way We Do Today

The love of money is the root of all evils.
1 Timothy 6:10, RSV

Chapter 13

Who Starts the Fads?

We are a long way from a healthful life today. We are eating many foods which are strange departures from the food God provides in nature. When our desire is to feed our family nourishing and well-balanced meals, how have we fallen into a pattern which is neither? How have we fallen into a trap of altered foods, sugared foods, and foods loaded with additives? We talk about raising healthy families, yet our nation spends an estimated $100,000,000,000 annually on health care. And Christians are very much a part of that statistic. Our failure to eat wisely and to be abundantly healthy is what I feel we must examine as closely and honestly as we do the other areas of our Christian lives.

My study leads me to believe that we have been deceived in one or more ways. Some of us have been misled by the spread of fads; others have believed unwarranted allegations against reliable nutritionists and biochemists; many of us have been given a preponderance of misinformation, even from impressive sources; and most of us have both seen and heard a great deal of misrepresentation. Beyond these, there are numerous cases in which important information concerning today's food has been withheld from us. And a few of us have been taken in by extreme and cultist diets. I believe that if we are aware of why we eat the way we do today, we can make a more informed and, therefore, a more honest evaluation of this area of our lives.

The field of nutrition has its share of quacks and faddists. This fact, unfortunately, is often used against nutritionists by those in other health-related fields who are neither students nor exponents of nutrition. However, this unhappy aspect must be kept in perspective. What field does not have a certain percentage of quacks and faddists? The medical profession certainly has a lamentably high percentage, but we do not dismiss all doctors because of the imposters, the poorly trained and dangerous among them. We should show the same discretion with nutritionists.

Nutrition, in the context in which I speak, is hardly a fad. The real fad, as I mentioned before, is that which man has contrived—the refined flours, the sugar, the overprocessed and convenience foods, as well as the unnatural methods used in farming and in raising animals. The twentieth century has brought unprecedented fads in foods which were never imagined by our forebears and certainly not intended by our Creator.

What About Fads?

Doctors, too, have started fads through the years. The most widespread one today is the panic over saturated fat, the rush for polyunsaturates, and the elimination of the egg. It seems to be out of hand, especially when biochemists and nutritionists tell us that a reasonable amount of saturated fat is essential to good health and strength and that the excessive use of polyunsaturates can cause problems.

There is no question that the average American diet is too high in saturated fat because the average American diet is a poor one. It is made up of an inordinate amount of meat from quickly and overly fattened livestock, ill-made gravies and sauces, sausages and luncheon meats in which the fat is disguised with coloring, pastries and convenience foods which are high in fat content, and quantities of fried foods. Furthermore, in many of these foods we find a poor quality of fat and sometimes fat which is overused and rancid. We cannot disregard the fact that excessive consumption of saturated fats can cause diverse problems, including indigestion. However, we should not look upon saturated fat as an evil, but rather as an essential to good health when consumed in sensible amounts. We need not become polyunsaturated fat faddists. Nor should we be influenced by the advertising of industries which are capitalizing on this fad.

Richard Passwater, a biochemist who is known in scientific circles for his research on cancer and heart disease, says he finds "the heavy promotion of polyunsaturates dangerous." He points out that "the American diet has increased its polyunsaturate content, and that heart disease incidence paralleled it. . . . polyunsaturated oils increased from 14.4 pounds per person in 1946 to 19.0 pounds per person 1963. Heart disease mortality kept pace with this increase." He maintains that "other dangers of excess polyunsaturates include nutritional muscular dystrophy, increased uric-acid levels (a factor in gout and possibly heart disease), increased incidence of gallstones, and under certain conditions even increased blood-cholesterol levels." [1]

Our nation's consuming concern with reducing the saturated fat content of foods has led to another experiment in altering animals. We learn from the *Wall Street Journal* that researchers at the University of California have developed polyunsaturated cows.[2] Cattle are fed special grain which delays the digestive processes by bypassing the stomach that normally turns grain into saturated fat. (Milk normally contains only 3% polyunsaturated fat.) The result of the new process is that steers produce meat and cows produce milk which are low in saturated fat. Controlled tests on students who consumed the polyunsaturated products showed a 14% lower serum-cholesterol than the students fed the same diet from normal animals. They say that the study has caused great excitement among the medical researchers at the university. At this time, FDA approval is still needed. A former FDA official is quoted as saying that the agency will have to be satisfied that flavor and storage problems won't develop. Let's hope the consideration will go beyond that. For instance, how good is short-circuiting the normal digestive process of an animal for the animal? And how good is its altered meat and milk for the human being over a period of years? There seems to be no end to trying to disrupt the balance of nature.

What About Eggs?

Nutritionists are constantly reminding us that the egg is a highly nutritious food and an important part of our diet. Many thousands of people, however, do not eat them, or they eat very few, because they are afraid of the saturated fat content. On an average, an egg actually contains six grams of fat of which four are polyunsaturated.[3] As concerns the saturated fat content of eggs, "eggs are particularly rich in lecithin, the very substance medical researchers have shown to be cholesterol controlling." [4] Cheraskin speaks of the "wisdom of nature. In nature we find carbohydrates with the vitamins and minerals, and we find cholesterol packaged with what is needed for it to be completely beneficial." Besides lecithin, an egg furnishes the following nutrients: high quality protein with important amino acids—lysine, leucine, isoleucine, methionine, threonine, tryptophan, phenylalanine, valine, arginine, and histidine. It has saturated and unsaturated fats, iron, phosphorous, trace minerals, and vitamin A, all the B vitamins, and vitamins D, E, and K. What a pity that the general public does not know the facts about eggs—especially when the cost of meat is so high.

What About Cholesterol?

Nonetheless, the all-consuming concerns of Americans today are cholesterol levels and avoiding saturated fats which they have been led to believe is the main culprit causing high cholesterol levels and, eventually, heart disease. Cheraskin points out that cholesterol is made from carbohydrates as well as fats.[5] Futhermore, we have recently been hearing a great deal more about sugar and the fact that, among the carbohydrates, it appears to be the major offender.

Passwater points out that many cholesterol tests have been misleading for two reasons: First of all, rabbits are usually used, and they are vegetarians and not equipped to handle dietary cholesterol; secondly, some tests are invalid because they use purified cholesterol crystals instead of natural food containing cholesterol. Another point he makes is that "wherever nature puts cholesterol, lecithin is there to keep it soluble in the blood." [6]

The fact many of us do not realize is that 80% of the cholesterol in our blood is manufactured within the body by the liver and other organs. One scientist tells us that "dietary cholesterol does not increase blood cholesterol; there is a feedback mechanism that adjusts the total body cholesterol amount to the amount we get from our food. When we eat more cholesterol we make less in our bodies." [7] And Cheraskin tells us that "Eliminating foods containing cholesterol from your diet can actually escalate a cholesterol problem since there is ample evidence that when a diet is deficient in pre-formed cholesterol, a complicated feedback system goes into operation which encourages the body to manufacture excess amounts of this substance." [8]

Dr. Michael DeBakey, the prominent heart surgeon, has said that he and his associates have found little relationship between diet, cholesterol levels, and progression in coronary disease. DeBakey has said, "Much to the chagrin of many of my colleagues who believe in this polyunsaturated fat and cholesterol business, we have put our patients on no dietary program and no anti-cholesterol medications. [9] The eminent Dr. Denton Cooley, Surgeon-in-Chief of the Texas Heart Institute, thinks that "there are too many faddists in medicine who put patients on strict low cholesterol programs." [10]

Probably the most important information the layman needs to know is that, first of all, both saturated and unsaturated fats are important to good health. And secondly, as Dr. Edward Pinckney, author of *The Cholesterol Controversy*, writes, "No matter what you have seen or heard to the contrary, few people realize that there has never been a proven, scientific relationship between the blood cholesterol levels and preventing heart disease." [11] Of further interest is that as of 1975, the National Heart and Lung Institute will provide more than $1,000,000 to three universities for the first year of study to determine whether there is a relationship between cholesterol levels and heart disease.

In order to better understand the proper cholesterol balance in the body, it is important that we learn as much as we can from biochemists and nutritionists working in this area. Significant discoveries are continually being made. For example, Dr. Constance Spittle of England and Professor Emil Ginter of Czechoslovakia have both found in their research that sufficient amounts of vitamin C in the diet can mean less cholesterol in the arteries. There is further evidence that the cholesterol problem is related to a lack of nutrients besides lecithin and vitamin C. These include nicotinic acid and grain and vegetable fiber which Cheraskin says are "cholesterol lowering agents and help the body to regenerate cholesterol levels." [12] In other words, we keep coming back to the fact that good health depends upon a proper balance of foods and complete nutrition.

What Should We Eat?

Where fats are concerned, we should eat a balance of good quality saturated fat and good quality unsaturated fat—and neither to excess; a 25% proportion of our diet is a reasonable amount of a total of both fats. Good quality unsaturated fat is found in the natural, unrefined vegetable oils. Good quality saturated fat is found in properly fed animals and pure dairy products. We must bear in mind that today most animals—cows, sheep, pigs, and chickens—have a great deal of fat on them because of the way they were raised. The animals our ancestors ate were much leaner. Wild animals that primitive people eat can be compared to our wild deer; venison is lean. These animals have more *un*saturated fat. The beef we get in our market today comes from cattle which have been quickly fattened in feed lots. Therefore, the meat, as well as the fat, is of a different composition. We are well-advised to eat lean meat; this is one of the reasons why organically fed animals are superior. When our economy caused many feed lots to close down for a time and some of us started getting meat from the pasture, we were better off than we knew. Also, if the economy has caused some of us to eat more fish, we are better off than we may realize. Beef is a good source of protein, but we overdo it in our country and deprive ourselves of the special nutrition, as well as the leanness, of fish. And eat eggs. Cheraskin says that we should eat one a day, two if we enjoy them. They furnish more nutrients per calorie than any other single food except milk.[13]

In summary, faddists and quacks do show up in the field of nutrition. They can be identified by their lack of extensive education in biochemistry and nutrition, by their recommendation of extreme and unbalanced diets, and by their unfounded claims. Unfortunately, many people have been misled by them, and this is one of the reasons why many eat the way they do today.

There is another reason, however, and a more important one, why we eat the way we do. We have yielded to the much more pervasive fads started by some powerful industries with particular economic interests and by some members of the medical profession with particular preoccupations.

Learning about and eating whole food in the form in which God provided it, and in the form in which families have consumed it for thousands of years, is *not* a fad. We must not allow ourselves or our children to be persuaded that it is.

Chapter 14

Misrepresentation and Misinformation

One source of misrepresentation of food products is advertising. This is especially true of advertising on television where a complete illusion can be communicated through a simple action or association. For example, strapping athletes and other heroes give the public the impression that they are great because of the refined cereal they eat. One advertisement uses a ball and chain to symbolize the burden of being overweight and shows how the ball and chain are removed by eating a certain refined cereal (plus, of course, a heaping teaspoon of sugar). Then we have the woman whose common sense tells her that if she eats a bowl of the advertised cereal she won't have to worry about vitamins all day!

One of the newer cereals, Buc Wheats, claims to be "high nutrition." We hear about its protein and vitamin-mineral value on television, but we do not hear about its other ingredients:

> Sugar
> Brown sugar syrup
> Malt syrup
> Artificial flavors
> Maple syrup
> Gum acacia
> BHT and other additives

Can it really be said that a cereal provides "high nutrition" when it contains chemicals and sweets which cause tooth decay and other problems?

Perhaps the advertisement which bothers me most is the one which shows a "home economist" who makes sure that her family drinks a substitute for fresh orange juice every morning because it is so nutritious. Furthermore, the viewer is supposed to be impressed by the fact that astronauts drink this substitute in space. The advertisement does not give us the list of ingredients in this mixture. The mixture, Tang, actually contains:

> Sugar
> Citric acid
> Calcium Phosphate (to regulate tartness and prevent caking)
> Gum Arabic (vegetable gum—provides body)
> Natural flavor
> Potassium Citrate (regulates tartness)
> Vitamin C
> Cellulose Gum (vegetable gum)
> Hydrogenated coconut oil
> Artificial flavor
> Artificial color
> Vitamin A
> BHT (a preservative)

We note that sugar is listed first. By law, ingredients must be listed according to their prevalance in the product.

My hope would be that although astronauts must drink artificial orange juice in space, they take advantage of pure fresh orange juice at home. The real thing has a great deal more nutrition to offer than just vitamin C. However, advertisers would have us believe that the manufacturer's substitute, with its assortment of sugars, chemical additives, and artificial flavor and color, is an equivalent substitute. We have a choice between nature's provisions and man's money-making, artificial imitations.

William Robbins, who has made a penetrating study and report on the food industry, tells us that we pay billions of dollars to be bombarded by advertising messages designed to persuade us that worse is really better.[1] He says that the food industry is a formidable concentration of power represented by lobbyists with strong political influence in Washington. The industry tells us that we are blessed with better food at lower costs than are people in any other country. Robbins asks, "Better than what?" To what can our food be compared when it is grown, processed, and impregnated with chemicals? Robbins says that more intelligent consumer buying can change the course of events. It seems obvious that not being misled by advertisements, coupled with taking time to read labels, would do much to bring about more intelligent consumer buying.

We need every reminder we can get to read labels. The following cartoon is one.

THE LOCKHORNS

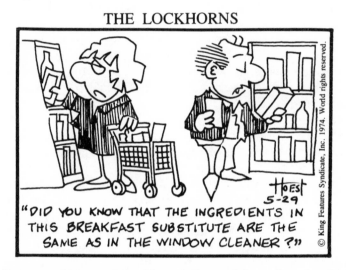

"DID YOU KNOW THAT THE INGREDIENTS IN THIS BREAKFAST SUBSTITUTE ARE THE SAME AS IN THE WINDOW CLEANER?"

Congratulations, Mr. Hoest! Everything that is done to alert us to the fact that we sometimes eat foodless foods is to be commended. An enormous amount of information and action is needed to counteract the billion dollar advertising program which reaches into every home and every mind with its misrepresentations.

Dr. Michael Jacobson[2] informs us that the breakfast cereal industry devotes about 13% of its income to advertising. This means that when we buy refined and sugared products, we help pay for misleading advertisements. Is this what we want to do?

Misinformation

Misinformation is another deception with which we must cope. There is no end to the misinformation on every subject in the world, but when it comes to nutrition, deception abounds at every turn and to the most extreme degrees. My book deals with misinformation in many forms, and to this I would like to add an example of the kind of false advice we can get from sources which sound authoritative. My example is an article entitled "Fast-Food Menus Get an 'A' for Nutrition in Professor's Study." The article reported on an account given by Howard Appledorf, an assistant professor at the University of Florida Institute of Food and Agricultural Sciences in the April, 1974, issue of *Food Technology*. The gist of the article was that Appledorf had found the staple menu of hamburger, French fries, vanilla shakes, and specialty items from big chains "nutritionally ideal." He observed that such a meal provides one-third of the recommended daily allowance of calories, protein, calcium, phosphorus, zinc, and copper. The article concluded that "overall, Mr. Appledorf believes that franchise fast-foods 'can be an acceptable source of nutrition and that nutritional labeling of fast foods should be encouraged.' "

There is no argument with the fact that every food possible should have nutritional labeling. (However, I doubt if that means anything to the average housewife, especially if the label capitalizes on the low and arbitrary figure of the RDA.) But the inference of the article is completely out of line with the opinions of doctors and nutritionists alike.

One illustration comes from a UPI report of an investigation made by Dr. Richard Bogg of Indiana.[3] Bogg compares youths in the Muncie area who have serious acne problems to a similar age group in Ireland who have beautiful complexions. The Muncie youths eat large quantities of hamburgers, French fries, and soft drinks, while the Irish youths do not frequent hamburger stands, do not snack, and definitely do not eat as many items that have been deep-fat fried.

A diet of hamburgers, French fries, shakes, or soft drinks is also out of line with the common-sense opinion of some laymen. Whereas these laymen may not be well enough informed to be critical of the use of refined flour in the hamburger bun, of the process of frying both the meat and potatoes, or of the fact that a soft drink has the approximate equivalent of five teaspoons of sugar and a milk shake of eight, they do know that the lack of green vegetable or salad and fruit keeps any lunch from being "nutritionally ideal." Yet, a professor in the Food and Agricultural Sciences at a university would make such a statement!

It is statements such as this which would indicate the grip of nutritional ignorance our nation is in; it also tells us what kind of nutrition is taught at some of our universities. Furthermore, this statement gives credence to the cases we hear about in which industry funds researchers to work in their interests. Such statements are invaluable to the fast-food industry and appeal highly to youth. And they are believed by adults who do not know better.

Another source of misinformation comes from our government itself. Its agencies have set up offices in various parts of the country which advertise over the radio that they are happy to supply you with facts on food; and they give a number of these "facts" over the air. Some of their statements are accurate and helpful. Others are not, nor can they be substantiated. Actually, some of them are propaganda for the views of the FDA upon which they are trying to legislate. The inaccurate statements are those which are based upon the arbitrary figure the FDA set for the recommended daily allowance; the figure is given as though it were scientifically proven, which it is not. Furthermore, their agencies equate whole-grain products with those made of "enriched" flour. Beyond this is their propaganda: the claim that taking food supplements without a doctor's advice is a form of self-medication, equating vitamins with drugs. They advise us to go to the doctor for advice on vitamins, thereby implying that doctors are trained in nutrition and qualified to advise us on it. Furthermore, they fail to warn us about sugar, including the fact that it is found in almost every package and jar in the supermarket. They fail, also, to warn us about foods which are disguised in one way or another to make them saleable.

One example of how the government instructs the nation to eat is the elaborate and colorful booklet it published as a guide. Its first page quotes Richard Nixon's message to Congress on May 6, 1969: "People must be educated in the choosing of proper foods. All of us ... must be reminded that a proper diet is a basic determinant of good health." The booklet was prepared by the U.S. Departments of Agriculture and Health, Education and Welfare *in cooperation with* the Grocery Manufacturers of America and the Advertising Council. The products of the Grocery Manufacturers and the messages of its advertisers are enough to tell us what kind of a guide to eating the government has published for us!

These are only a few examples of the misrepresentation and misinformation meted out to us in various ways, but they are indicative of what is happening. Industry continues to alter food and spend billions to tell us how nutritious its concoctions are, and government condones a great deal of this. It is no wonder that the Christian has been misled or that some of us eat the way we do. We need not continue to be deceived, however, and we need not give silent approval to the practices which displease us today in either government or industry—even though they are astronomically wealthy allies.

Charles Spurgeon reminded us, "He who loves truth must hate every false way." [4] Matthew 10:16 says, "Be wise as serpents" (RSV). Are we justified in believing that these admonitions pertain to everything in the Christian life except God's most tangible gift to us—our bodies?

Chapter 15

Withheld Information

Withheld information is one of the most direct reasons why some of us eat the way we do. Although we realize that large corporations sometimes withhold information from the public, we would expect that those in the food industry would not do this, especially when it concerns people's health. My studies reveal, however, that some of them suppress a great deal of information. One has only to read a few of the investigative and well-documented reports recently written to be alarmed. Too often projects supported by chemical, food, and agricultural industries appear to be independent and unbiased. Actually, these projects and the reports on them may be attempts on the part of the industries to disseminate misleading material and suppress information which would expose or raise questions concerning the truth. They suppress information by publishing attacks on their critics, by putting reports unfavorable to their own product on a "not recommended list," or by using all sorts of devious methods to keep information damaging to their product out of print altogether.

Withheld Information on Additives

Beatrice Trum Hunter lists examples of organizations which act as propaganda agencies for their own particular interests: American Dairy Association, National Dairy Council, American Meat Institute, National Livestock and Meat Board, Cereal Institute, Wheat Flour Institute, Wheat and Wheat Foods Foundation, and the Sugar Research Foundation, Inc. Two cases which bear out what she says involve William Longgood's *The Poisons in Your Food* and Rachel Carson's *Silent Spring*.

Withheld Information on Pollution

Promptly after publication of *The Poisons in Your Food*, a scathing review of it appeared in *Science* (April, 1960) by Dr. William J. Darby, a prominent nutritionist. Dr. Darby's research has been supported by funds from the Nutrition Foundation (which, as Mrs. Hunter has told us, is funded by the largest food processors and refiners in America), as well as by grants from manufacturers of synthetic vitamins, drugs, and chemicals. Dr. Darby's review was promptly reprinted by a chemical trade association and distributed widely to newspaper editors throughout the country. The Nutrition Foundation sent the review and a letter to librarians, along with another unfavorable review written by its executive director at the time, Dr. Charles Glen King. How many librarians were aware of the fact that the materials discrediting *The Poisons in Your Food* were sent out by an organization sponsored by the food industry?

When the publication of Rachel Carson's *Silent Spring* threatened to upset the pesticide industry, the Nutrition Foundation, together with the Manufacturing Chemists' Association, put together a "fact kit" on *Silent Spring*. The kit consisted of a defense of chemical pesticides prepared by the New York State College of Agriculture, included a letter signed by the Nutrition Foundation's president, Dr. King, who labeled the book unscientific and the author a "professional journalist—not a scientist in the field of her discussion," and also contained the reprinted book reviews, all derogatory, including those written by the Nutrition Foundation's Drs. Frederick Stare and William Darby.

Happily, suppressive forces don't always win out. *Silent Spring* won eight awards and was a history-making best seller. It was given acclaim by distinguished individuals and by book reviewers. The *Chicago Daily News* said of Rachel Carson: "Miss Carson is a scientist and is not given to tossing serious charges around carelessly ... *Silent Spring* may well be one of the great and towering books of our time. This book is a *must* reading for every responsible citizen." Justice William O. Douglas called *Silent Spring* "The most important chronicle of this century for the human race." Yet the Nutrition Foundation and Manufacturing Chemists' Association did their utmost to discredit Miss Carson and quash her book!

Withheld Information on Sugar

Another situation which may shake our comfortable illusions about the motives of the food industry involves Dr. John Yudkin. Yudkin, author of *Sweet and Dangerous*, describes his collision with the sugar industry. He tells of an international conference on nutrition at which he was an honored speaker. In his speech he mentioned his theories and research on the harm of sugar consumption. Sometime later, when the secretary of the international organization sponsoring the conference was organizing the conference papers for publication, he asked Yudkin if he would mind deleting his reference to sugar. Yudkin refused and said that the only alternative would be to omit his paper from the book. The secretary omitted his paper. This is an example of the influence of the food industry. We are left to conclude that money speaks louder than health.

Crime Against the Food Law

There was a noble and learned gentleman in the early 1900s who could predict the future of any nation whose foods and drugs were not kept free of any adulteration and misbranding and whose manufacturers were not dedicated to producing the natural, wholesome foods which insure the health of its people. This man is remembered with honor by those who work diligently to reverse the course of adulteration and fabrication and the less than honest advertising which now exists in much of the food and beverage industry.

This man was Dr. Harvey W. Wiley, and he was founder and head of the Bureau of Chemistry which was established in 1907 and empowered by Congress to legislate, to inspect, and to take the offenders of the food and drug laws to court.[1] Wiley and his bureau proceeded conscientiously and boldly to publish bulletins on the deleterious physical effects of certain chemicals in use then and to enforce the law to the letter. This incensed some of the large manufacturers of beverages and foods. Months of battling in courts and lobbying in Washington ensued. It all ended in the suppression of Wiley's bulletins and, eventually, in the demise of the Bureau of Chemistry. Wiley was forced to resign from the bureau in order to be able to speak out in public and to the Congress. He wrote a book telling the whole story of how protective laws were scuttled from within the government. His manuscript disappeared while at the printer's. Ten years later, Wiley completed another book entitled *The History of Crime Against the Food Law* which was published in 1929. William Dufty writes that the book, which looked like a best seller, disappeared rapidly from bookstores and libraries. "Yet, no letters were received from the readers, no congratulations, no kudos, and virtually no reviews. The books kept on disappearing, yet copies could not be found anywhere." [2]

Had Wiley's scientific expose not been withheld, suppressed, and quashed, stories of attempted suppressions like those of William Longgood and Rachel Carson, and the many others which have been suppressed, might not exist for the telling today. Controls could already have been set and enforced, all new information could be gratefully received, examined, and acted upon by the government, and you and I might not be the victims of withheld information today.

The Federation of Homemakers' statement is that they are "Dedicated to furthering the philosophy of Doctor Harvey W. Wiley, father of our first Pure Food and Drug Act."

Chapter 16

Extreme and Cultist Diets

We are seeing an unprecedented trend towards exotic and extreme diets among a surprising number of young people in our country today. Sometimes the diet is part of a search for a way of life; often, however, it is not. One of the extreme diets we are seeing is total vegetarianism.

Many people on a vegetarian diet say they feel so much better at first. They should; it is probably the first time in their lives that they are not eating so many worthless foods and are benefiting from real foods like whole grains, nuts, seeds, sprouts, fresh vegetables, and fruits. As time goes on, however, many seem to become less active and do not look as well, and it is often the second generation which does not look as strong, especially if they and their parents are not lacto-vegetarians (those who eat dairy products as well as vegetables). In any event, some vegetarians can not know for years whether they have actually maintained a healthy body on their restricted diet.

I have heard a number of nutritionists say that it is possible to stay well as a vegetarian if one gets enough high-quality protein, but this is difficult to do. It is especially difficult for vegetarians to get enough protein into their growing children. Consequently, as a rule they have less resistance to disease and are deficient in amino acids. One case cited at a convention of the International Academy of Metabology was a young woman who showed a marked deficiency in amino acids and was getting only 44% of the calories she needed. To learn about adequate protein intake in their diets, I suggest that vegetarians read *Diet for a Small Planet* by Frances Moore Lappé and *Recipes for a Small Planet* by Ellen Buchman Ewald.

Some vegetarians and advocates of cultists diets have their own health food stores and restaurants, and many of these businesses are clean, well-managed, and reliable. Others are run by people who look as though they take India very seriously, including its lack of sanitation; they offer literature and lessons on cultic practices. Many, however, provide books based on sound nutrition.

The Zen Macrobiotic diet, which is one the current fascinations, actually has little connection with the Zen Buddhist monks in Japan who were known for their health and long lives. The Macrobiotic diet was devised by George Ohsawa and can be very dangerous. It consists of seven steps, starting with rice and a little water. After that the strict followers progress to a diet including other foods but little water; therein, apparently, lies the danger. Dr. Ruther Leverton, who is science advisor to the U.S. Department of Agriculture, has cited some of the possible results from an extreme Macrobiotic diet: scurvy, anemia, emaciation due to starvation, loss of kidney function due to restricted fluid intake, other forms of malnutrition, and some fatalities.[1]

Besides vegetarianism and strange diets, we are constantly hearing of new diets to lose weight—most of them extreme. It is hard to pick up a magazine which doesn't think it has the best. And we are bombarded by advertising, even on television, trying to persuade us to take up a certain system. Unfortunately, sometimes these diets are promoted by people whose primary motivation is to capitalize on this, the most obvious manifestation of our poor dietary habits. Undoubtedly, because of the way we have abused our bodies, many Americans should lose weight. It is crucial, however, in designing our diets that we do so with more knowledge and utmost attention to good nutrition.

Young people today are looking for harmony within themselves, harmony with others and with the universe. They are trying to realize these fundamental relationships through experimenting with new life styles; included in these new styles are various means of meditation and alternative ways of growing, preparing, and selecting foods. Young people would not have been left to rely upon their own ingenuity alone, however, or upon the religions of Asia if we as Christians had ourselves fully appreciated the value of our extraordinary bodies and allowed room for our own exuberance.

Both the value of the body and the freedom of the spirit are central to our Christian tradition. But we certainly haven't communicated this through our Sunday schools or our homes, nor have we offered it in a convincing way as we rush about and gulp down lifeless food.

We must understand our own failure before we criticize young people for attempting to find meaning and vitality elsewhere. Our faith offers all they are searching for and, of course, a tremendous amount more, but they could hardly know this from looking at us.

PART 5

Family Nutrition

Train up a child in the way he should go, and when he is old he will not depart from it.

Proverbs 22:6, RSV

Chapter 17

Nutrition

If we are to face reality about wholeness in the Christian life, we will look upon the care of the body as one dimension of it. The reality is that man is a food-dependent creature, and he cannot be what God intended physically and mentally if he is not nourished as God intended him to be. Dr. Roger Williams asserts that ulcers and diseases of the circulatory system, diarrhea, constipation, and alcoholism may be due to faulty nutrition.[1] Dr. Weston Price, in his global observations, corroborates what nutritionists and biochemists have been trying to tell us about the relationship between poor nutrition (our departure from natural and balanced foods) and the many degenerative diseases which plague our nation.[2] As we have also heard, psychiatrists and other experts are discovering how much nutrition has to do with mental and emotional problems. As Christians do we give serious thought to what we eat?

Relation Between What We Eat and Our Health

When we understand that our cells depend upon what we feed them, we understand why their malfunction brings about or contributes to most of our ills. One way, perhaps, to start giving serious thought to what we eat is to review a few of the processes of the body which depend upon what we put into it. For instance, when we say that every cell in our body depends upon proper nourishment daily, we mean specifically that the tissues of the stomach and intestines need the nourishment so that proper digestion and elimination take place. Our bones need nourishment, for they are alive too. Biochemists have found that minerals are constantly leaving and entering the bones. If our bones were dead, they would never heal when broken. We have to nourish the cells in the walls of our arteries and veins, our heart muscle cells, and our hormone-producing cells. What we eat plays a definite part in maintaining the health of our gums and teeth, our skin, and our hair. What we eat affects our endocrine balance, our brain, and our nervous system. Every bodily process depends upon proper nourishment; every cell in the body must be furnished with everything it needs, which means that if certain cells are not given what they need, the bodily process may be impaired. Dr. Cheraskin explains that there is no body activity in which nutrition is not involved and, further, that all nutrients are interrelated. "In other words," he says "the optimal functioning of every single nutrient is dependent upon the presence of every other essential nutrient." [3]

Many of us start the day with a piece of white-bread toast or a sweet roll, maybe a bowl of refined cereal with sugar on it, or a breakfast substitute of sugar, flour, chemical additives, artificial flavor and coloring, and coffee. Some settle for coffee alone. Many of us grab a quick sandwich for lunch—often two thick sides of a bun or bread made with refined flour and a thin fried meat patty or some other kind of filling, a sugared dessert, and plenty of coffee. Some skip lunch altogether. This is the way we dash off, offering the Lord our inadequately fueled, poorly nourished bodies to do whatever job He has set before us. We would not think of giving our car an inadequate amount or a poor grade of gas and oil with which to do a job, yet we are not at all careful about the fuel we give our own bodies. We have lost sight of the fact that how we nourish our bodies is a part of our stewardship as Christians.

Another illustration of man's inconsistency in relating what he eats to how he functions is my father's favorite story. He told about the owner of a stable of race horses who made sure every day that his horses were being fed exactly the right food: certain foods for health, for endurance, for good coats, for eyesight, for muscle tone, for mental alertness, and so forth. Then the owner would go home and throw anything into his own stomach! That is how much sense we show in our eating. We know that what we feed our dog is most important to his health, and then we call people who eat properly "food faddists."

Our Nutritional Illiteracy

We eat what we like; we diet for awhile if we want to lose weight; we call almost any kind of variety a "well-balanced meal"; and the truth is that many of us really do not know enough about nutrition to have any idea what a well-balanced meal is. Dr. George M. Briggs, Professor of Nutrition at the University of California at Berkeley, claims that the nation's nutritional illiteracy results in annual costs of about $30,000,-000,000 in health care, absenteeism, etc., which he says is equivalent to nearly one-third of our health bill and one-fourth of our food bill.

We do not know whether we are feeding the cells of our body properly. Then we blame everything else when we get sick—everything except what we have been eating all our life. Louis Pasteur started the germ theory, and we took it up from there. But we forget that Louis Pasteur also spoke of the "terrain," as he called it, from which we pick up or do not pick up a germ. How is our resistance? That is the major question and the major reason for being sure we are furnishing every cell in our body what it needs.

Leonardo da Vinci said, "Nature never breaks its laws," and that is accurate. God does not break His physical laws any more than He breaks His spiritual laws, and this is why I feel the lack of taking a stand for good nutrition is an indictment against the Christian community. We are very conscious of God's spiritual laws, yet most of us give no heed at all to His physical laws for the health of our bodies. The church, or the Christian community at large, has never, to my knowledge, spoken out on the fact that we are to respect and take care of the temple of God in the way God intended with His natural, unadulterated provisions. Certainly Christians cannot be expected to dictate specifically on diet, but we can speak out on the importance of proper nutrition and our responsibility as stewards of God's provisions for our bodies as well as our souls. After all, we speak out on all other areas of stewardship.

In this latter part of the twentieth century, we have even more demands upon our constitution. We are victims of physical degeneration which has changed man's perspective and evaluation. We are told that nothing could affect an entire nation more than its diet—a generation by generation deterioration due to cells not getting what they need. We are also being told that today fewer and fewer American families escape mental trouble and that what used to be considered "normal" may now simply mean "ideal"—a tragic disintegration of mental health standards. Furthermore, we are faced with pollutions our forefathers never knew.

The pollutions our bodies must withstand today require even greater bodily defenses in order to combat them. The nutritional experts tell us that ample vitamin supplementation helps to meet this crisis. On top of pollutions, our nervous systems must withstand the avalanche of changes which confront us, changes in every facet of our lives which demand constant, and sometimes drastic, personal readjustments. In his book *Future Shock*, Alvin Toffler quotes Kenneth Boulding as saying that there has been more change during the period of our lifetime than there has been in the entire span of years between Christ's time on earth and today—imagine this if you can. Mr. Toffler goes on to say:

> The disturbing fact is that the vast majority of people, including educated and otherwise sophisticated people, find the idea of change so threatening that they attempt to deny its existence. Even many people who understand intellectually that change is accelerating, have not internalized that knowledge, do not take this critical social fact into account in planning their own personal lives.[4]

Realizing all that our minds, nerves, and bodies must withstand, there seems to be no alternative to coming to grips with God's natural order for health if we are to survive with strong bodies and minds.

In view of the overwhelming evidence accrued on how far afield we have strayed from God's natural provisions for us and the enormous price in health we are paying for this transgression, are we prepared to do something about it? If so, we must start with ourselves. We must approach the changeover of our family diet intelligently and patiently. We must learn more about nutrition; we must learn how to market—what to buy, what to avoid—and we must improve our cooking methods where needed.

Prenatal Nutrition

The outlook is not bleak for the conscientious. The nutritionists whom I have heard tell us not only that we can be healthier ourselves through proper nutrition, but that by feeding ourselves properly, there can be a generation by generation restoration; this is encouraging news.

Dr. Roger Williams says:

> If a mother is not completely healthy and well nourished in every respect, she may fail to furnish the embryo with the best nutrition. In this case all sorts of difficulties—major and minor—may arise, depending upon what nutritional items are in short supply and how great are the shortages. . . . Cells may be very well nourished or they may be 'starved' ever so slightly and with respect to one or more of many nutrients. Nature has provided in a most intricate manner that growing embryonic cells can get—to a reasonably satisfactory degree—everything they need, provided the mother eats wisely. If she tries to subsist on anything less than a nutritious diet, the embryonic cells are bound to be starved in many ways. . . . Mothers need to be nourished with more than ordinary care if the cells which make up the growing embryo are furnished nutrition at a *high level* of efficiency.[5]

Obviously, both parents should be healthy. Proper nutrition is also advised for the father long before conception. Thus, the health of the child starts with the parents. Dr. Weston Price has seen conclusively what good nutrition means to stature, health, strength, and teeth, but he has also seen the correlation between poor prenatal nutrition and deformities, and physical, mental, and moral deterioration.[6] On our trips to many parts of the world we were impressed that primitive tribes, and the not-so-primitive, were very careful about prenatal nutrition and special nutrition during lactation. Price cited a number of strong tribes in which girls were put on special diets before marriage in order to be most physically fit for childbearing. The wisdom of the savage—that we might be as wise!

Nutrition and the Baby

The full cycle of life, then, involves nutrition. Let us start with the baby's nutrition today.

One of the best things to happen in our country in the last decade is the return to natural childbearing and breast feeding. We can thank the young parents of this generation for taking this far more desirable course. Breast milk is the only perfect food for the newborn babe—how could anyone question it? At a seminar of the International College of Applied Nutrition, Dr. Elie A. Shneour, author of the book *Malnutrition and Brain Development*, said, "Human milk is an important substance for the human species. Its combination of protein and minerals are ideal and quite different from cow's milk." Dr. Shneour quoted Dr. H. K. Waller of England as suggesting that since the dominant factor of human growth is the development of the brain, then it is probable that the human milk composition is specifically related to rapid growth of the brain.

In any event, mothers who conscientiously breast-feed their babies need not be concerned with all the inconveniences and hazards of bottle feeding. Neither need they be concerned with the physical problems thousands of babies on formulas have—possible inaccuracies in the proportions of ingredients in the formula, including the addition of dextrose, and the possibility of colic due to the lack of enzymes in pasteurized milk, as well as many other problems formulas present. We cannot outwit nature; God's provisions are ideal.

The next step in infant feeding is the introduction of solid food, and this deserves the greatest care.

The baby food industry is the second most profitable business in the United States. It does $400,000,000 worth of business a year while babies in this country eat 150,000,000,-000 pounds of commercial baby foods a year, according to the opening chapter of *The Natural Baby Food Cookbook* by Margaret Elizabeth Kenda and Phyllis S. Williams.[7] They also tell us that if we feed our babies commercially packed jars of baby food, we are depriving them of the best available nutrition and may be causing lifetime feeding problems because they are not introduced to the variety of flavors and substances which bring strength and health. Kenda and Williams tell us that convenience baby foods cost more than natural home cooking and taste flat and dull. They say that making baby foods yourself takes little time, small effort, routine equipment, and can be accomplished with only a fraction of the expense. As they express it: "Your own good cooking can help give your child the most precious gift of love: the best physical and mental health."[8]

When you give your baby commercial baby foods, you are giving him the adulteration of processed food, additives, inferior foods masked with salt, sugar, and MSG. *The Natural Baby Food Cookbook* tells us that water is the major ingredient in about 40% of multiple varieties of baby foods, and the foods are stretched with sugar and starch. An example of what a mother is likely to find is even in a "High Meat Dinner" which is apt to "contain such additives as oat flour, wheat flour, cornstarch, tapioca starch, vegetable oils, dry whey, 'flavoring' and other starches and salts, to the point of making one shudder at the very idea of what 'Low Meat Dinner' might be."[9]

Modified starches are to be avoided, anyway, because of the evidence of their indigestibility. Kenda and Williams tell us that Dr. Thomas A. Anderson resigned his post as chief of the Heinz Nutritional Research Laboratory because the company would not act on his recommendation that modified starches be removed from baby food.[10] This adds one more to the hundreds of available concrete evidences that industry's goal is based on profit, not the nation's health. It is also superb evidence of the stand an individual of conscience can take.

Kenda and Williams put the case of natural foods versus altered foods into focus for us when they inform us that baby meats contain five times more salt than fresh meat and that commercially strained vegetables have been known to have as much as sixty times the salt of fresh vegetables. Sufficient salt (sodium) for infants occurs naturally in milk, in many vegetables, in meat, fish, and cheeses, so your baby will get enough without adding more.[11] We have already seen in previous chapters that natural sugars occur in vegetables and fruits in the amount intended for us to assimilate and with the accompanying nutrients and fiber given us by God. We also know that proteins and nutritious starches convert into glucose for our nourishment and a balanced metabolism. What we do not want our babies to have is additional processed, concentrated 100% sugar manufactured by man. We need not be told the physical dangers which lie ahead for infants who are improperly fed and whose poorly educated palates will dictate their choice of diet for the rest of their lives.

Nutrition and Youth

If a growing youngster always has good food in his home —that is, unadulterated food, whole-grain products, and so forth—his taste will be developed for it; other things will taste insipid in comparison. Dr. Roger Williams says:

> Since good nutrition fosters good nutrition, it becomes obvious why nutrition in young children is so important. If they are well nourished from the start, their regulatory mechanisms develop well, the working of their body wisdom approaches perfection, and they may go through life without ever suffering from the ills associated with malnutrition. . . . If you want your child not to overeat on sweets, feed him nutritiously. It is an established fact that a properly nourished child will automatically regulate his eating habits well. A deficient diet causes an over-consumption of sugar.[12]

If for a time he seems to reject that on which he has been raised, he at least has the benefit of a healthier body because of good eating habits at home, and he will return to them eventually. "Train up a child in the way he should go, and when he is old he will not depart from it" (Prov. 22:6). I can say from my experience that our three children, all now grown, are not pop drinkers (they were given fruit juices and milk while growing up), they do not like many sweets or too many carbohydrates, and they all eat natural foods by choice—even after going through the rigors of poor food while away at school and in spite of the bad eating habits of some of their peers.

We are hearing more about the fact that under-achievers and sometimes those with more serious problems are children who are not nutritiously fed. The lack of the nutrients they need for every cell in their body shows up in unexpected ways. It is our real responsibility to feed them what they need. Dr. Hugh

W. S. Powers, Jr., of Dallas, a physician of twenty years' experience with children, says, "The correct dietary measures improve the behavior and scholastic achievement of children.... For a child to think well he must have the right food.... Too often the psychological environment is blamed instead of the internal environment."

If our doctors have not studied nutrition and do not have a nutritionist (not a dietician) on their staff, we should find a good nutritionist and get expert advice. Our children undoubtedly need vitamin-mineral supplements, and if we cannot find a nutritionist, we will have to figure it out ourselves after studying some books on the subject. However, it is important that the child does not think the supplements take the place of his meals—a supplement is a supplement—his meals, properly prepared nutritious meals, are most important, including an adequate breakfast.

We often encounter problems in trying to get youngsters to eat differently from their peers. However, don't we experience this in other areas as well? If Christian parents are willing to stand firm in other areas of their children's lives, they can certainly be firm on the food issue for valid reasons. And these reasons should be explained to the child. It is easier today than it was ten and twenty years ago because it ties in with the ecology movement which is the big thing with young people whom children want to emulate. Furthermore, their peers may be very interested in your children's sandwiches made of whole or sprouted grains and the other surprises which make up a truly nutritious lunch pail. And, by the way, a lunch pail with nutritious food in it is far superior to what the child would be served by the school or buy on his own.

One thing for certain, your children's peers will rush to refrigerators filled with fruit juices, fresh lemonade, and fresh fruit punches; I know this from experience. It is shocking how many children are refreshed daily with artificial drinks from packages. The Bible says, "Whatever you do, work at it with all your heart, as working for the Lord, not for men" (Col. 3:23). Isn't it rather foolish, when one can serve one's family and friends lovely, wholesome, fresh juice from God-given fruit containing natural fructose and packed with vitamins and other essential properties, to serve, instead, pitchers of Kool-Aid:

"100% Sugar-Sweetened Imitation Lemonade Mix with Vitamin C" made from "Sugar, citric acid (provides tartness), gum arabic (vegetable gum), monosodium phosphate (controls acidity), natural lemon flavor, lemon juice dried with corn syrup solids, partially hydrogenated soybean and cotton seed oil, Vitamin C, glyceryl lacto stearate (emulsifier), mono- and diglycerides (emulsifiers), artificial color, BHA (preserves freshness)"? (wording from package). Is this serving lemonade "as to the Lord" or "for men"?

Christian families can take heart from an article which appeared in the *National Observer,* entitled "A Study That Explodes Old Logic," and subtitled "Children Turn to Drugs to Please Their Mod, Liberal-Minded Parents." The study, as one would expect, was comprehensively done from an interview with Richard H. Blum, Stanford University psychologist, top authority on drug misuse and consultant to the White House Special Action Office in Drug Abuse Prevention. The article points up the interesting findings on why youths are apt to take up drugs; it categorizes them as "low risk" and "high risk" families.

> Low risk families tended generally to venerate the "God-Country-family" creed. More often than high-risk families, low-risk families professed the importance of disciplining children "a lot" while still "attending to the child's preferences." Low-risk families tended to make basic decisions about the children's friends, food, study habits, church attendance, and bedtime longer than high-risk parents did. More often than high-risk couples, low-risk parents attended church and expressed satisfaction at the way they had raised their offspring.

So Christian discipline with love, fairness, and the parents' example still holds good. And good nutrition should surely be one of the basic disciplines.

"Train up a child in the way he should go, and when he is old he will not depart from it." And he will be the healthier adult for it.

The nutritional movement has gained impetus along with ecology, which is good. This makes nutritious food at home much easier for the senior high and college age group to accept. Also, the fact that health food stores, health food restaurants, and health food bars are cropping up all over, many of which are run by your children's peers, makes the transition for families with college age youth much easier. Some youth might even think the family is finally showing common sense!

The movement on the college campuses is a boon. The hardest part about sending our young people away to school and college some years back was the diet to which they had to submit. Today it is the high school and college student who has spearheaded the drive for pure foods. Some western universities are meeting the demand for experimental courses on organic gardening and organic cooking. Some have had seminars to evaluate processed foods, vitamins, additives, and naturally occuring toxicants in foods. Group organic cooking is becoming popular on college campuses today, and an increasing number of universities, including the University of California, Brandeis, Harvard, MIT, and Yale, serve organic meals. Albert Dobie, director of Yale University's dining halls, said that Adelle Davis was part of the reason for young people's awareness of good nutrition. He also said that "starchy diets that generations of collegians complained about are no more" and that he has noticed a real decrease in dessert consumption and a corresponding increase in demand for fresh fruit instead of cake and pie.[13]

This is good news to the family that does eat nutritious foods as well as to those who want to make the change. One wonders how many Christians sit on the Board of Regents and other advisory or governing councils of schools and colleges or how many faculty members there are who could be an influence for better nutrition in their establishments of learning?

Nutrition and the Patient

Another family concern when it comes to nutrition is the recuperating patient, no matter what age. As one biochemist has said, a nutritionist is more important at this time than a nurse. A patient needing to overcome the toxicity and other effects of drugs upon the body, as well as needing every available nutrient for healing and gaining strength, must be consuming the foods and supplements which promote recovery. The doctor may prescribe a general diet, and he often does not distinguish between the more nutritious and the less nutritious foods. For example, he prescribes bread and cereal as though they all did the same thing for the body. The truth of the matter is that there is a vast difference in what some breads and cereals do for the body. And this goes right down the line with other foods. In my experience with the recuperation of people of all ages, I find that because doctors are not trained in nutrition, they do not as a rule specifically check, much less keep track of, what a patient is consuming from the nutritional standpoint. I have even known cases when the doctor has prescribed a high-protein diet and never inquired how many grams the patient actually consumed, twenty-five or seventy-five. So, unless you have a capable nutritionist to advise you, the burden is on you to know the right kind of body-building food and supplements which will help overcome the effects of drugs, promote healing, and bring complete recovery.

A New Start for the Family

Starting a new regime in a family is going to take thought, study, and a right approach. The baby is no problem—babies want to do what comes naturally. It is always rewarding to be able to start with a baby and watch him develop a fine sense of taste. This has been my happy experience, and our children, now grown, all eat well, cook well, love wholesome food, and concoct their own recipes. It may take time to convert the rest of the family since industry has perverted their tastes, but they will be won over gradually as you discover together the savoriness of natural foods and understand what great things pure foods do for the body, nervous system, and mind. Other foods actually do become dull and tasteless when palates are reeducated to nature's treasures. Beatrice Trum Hunter has a helpful chapter on the subject, "You're Convinced, How Do You Convert Your Family?" in her book entitled *The Natural Foods Primer*.

One of the assets of reforming our eating habits is that it gets us out of the menu-planning ruts most of us get into all too easily. When we think of nutritional meals, we immediately open up new vistas and are in for all sorts of new taste treats—interesting twists to old dishes that make them taste better and new foods which redeem our menus.

Chapter 18

Marketing

To market healthfully we must market suspiciously—sad, but true. Any other approach would be naive. And one word we have to be suspicious of is "nutritious." Nutritious is the big word today; it is being pushed hard, and many manufacturers overdo it. The word is flaunted about to sell every kind of inferior product. In order to be good stewards, we need to know what is actually nutritious and what is not. We must also be careful about products which claim to be "natural" or "organic"; deceivers are playing their game with these words, too. We must know our way around the marketplace, we must read all labels carefully, and we must use reliable health food stores or other sources of natural and organically grown produce.

All we need nutritionally is available, but we must market with care. You will probably still shop in the usual markets, but you will also find yourself going to health food stores for many items. In the supermarket you will learn where the merchandise and fresh produce you want can be found, and you will also find that you wheel your cart right by many sections that no longer interest you. You are now looking for real food, not foodless food or partial food. You will frequent health food stores and discover the kinds of foods which now interest you—organically grown vegetables and meat, certified raw milk, good yogurts, fertile eggs, whole-grain products, seeds, and many other items. Some health food stores are better than others, of course, so visit several. Only a few have access to fresh produce. Actually, I don't like referring to these stores as health food stores because the designation "health food" is a misnomer. They are stores that sell natural foods which are healthful. It would be more correct to label some of the shelves in supermarkets "unnatural foods," "foodless foods," "altered foods," or "partial foods."

Fruits and Vegetables ·

When marketing for fruits and vegetables, buy those from organic farms if possible. Check the classified telephone directory under "Health Food Stores"; they sometimes describe what produce they carry. Also check the advertisements in magazines carried in health food stores. *The Organic Directory* is a directory for organic food sources and is prepared by Rodale Press, Inc., Emmaus, Pennsylvania, 18049. It tells what to look for in marketing for organic produce and gives an extensive list of farmers' markets, natural foods stores, organic growers, and organic food cooperatives by location.

Otherwise, take as much care as possible in picking out fruits and vegetables in the supermarket. Ordinarily we are taught to choose vegetables with deep coloring. However, we can no longer always go by this rule because industry deceives us by making some vegetables and fruits appear ripe when they are not—sometimes they even overdo the coloring. Most tomatoes we are eating now are not ripened on the vine, but are picked in southern climates and artificially treated to appear ripened. This is done by spraying them with ethylene gas in special gas chambers. Both from the viewpoint of taste and nutrition, Dr. Jean Mayer tells us, "such a tomato is inferior to the one which is ripened on the vine." [1] Unfortunately, the same process is used on some of the other fruits and vegetables such as citrus fruits and celery. Often the paler fruit or the less white celery, especially pascal, is superior because it has not seen the gas chamber.

Almost all fruit is picked when green. Some are picked so prematurely that they never do get ripe and sweet; they become moldy instead. I have had this happen so often with honeydew melons that I seldom take a chance on them anymore. Pineapples are also often picked so prematurely that you find them spoiled before they are ripe.

We will also remember that most vegetables and fruits on the general market have been subjected to plenty of chemical fertilizers and pesticides. Residues can be absorbed through the roots of the plants and have been found on their skins. Wax and coloring matter may also be used to make fresh produce more eye-appealing, such as on apples, plums, pears, peppers, carrots, cucumbers, eggplant, and potatoes. Potatoes are sometimes treated with chemicals to slow down sprouting and deceive us about their age. Other chemicals are sometimes used to coat vegetables to retard decay. As long as the Department of Agriculture sanctions this dishonesty, as indeed it must for it allows it, and as long as the public trustingly accepts the present standards of agriculture, you and I often really cannot know what we are buying.

The rules our grandparents depended upon to tell good produce can no longer be applied in many cases. If we do not have access to the produce from organic farms, we would do well to find out what we can about the sources our markets use. In season some markets deal with local farmers whose produce may not be as heavily dosed with chemical fertilizers and pesticides or subject to some of the other ills of mass production. The main rule to follow is to be sure of freshness and not buy fruits or vegetables with bruises, shrunken spots, discoloration, skin punctures, or limpness.

The sooner fresh produce is eaten after picking, the better. Happiness is the family with its own garden!

If we cannot obtain fresh produce in the market or from our garden, we have the choice of frozen or canned. Frozen produce is preferable although not ideal; it does have a few drawbacks. Some manufacturers claim to freeze their produce right at the field which, of course, saves nutrients. Most, however, cart it to plants, and the produce may wait around several days. This is also true in canning. Sometimes the produce is sprayed with chemicals to keep it fresh and to keep those discerning bugs away. Another drawback is that the produce is blanched for five minutes to destroy certain enzymes and there can be another vitamin loss in this procedure. Finally, 10% of the nutritional value is lost in defrosting, so it is important not to let frozen foods defrost before cooking. Sometimes frozen goods are thawed and refrozen in handling in shipment. For this reason do not buy packages which are frosty on the outside; sometimes a little pressure with the fingers will let you feel or hear whether it is frosty on the inside, too. However, frozen food does bring us fresh produce the year around and is superior to canning.

In canning, the manufacturer often introduces additives. Furthermore, the extreme heat used in canning causes more loss of nutrients, while the changes in the color, texture, and flavor of many vegetables makes the product inferior.

Dairy Products

When marketing for dairy products, if it is impossible to purchase certified or licensed raw milk, buy the freshest. The cartons are dated in most states. Buy natural cheeses and the purest butter which is freshly churned from sweet cream and has natural coloring and no additives except salt. Read the labels carefully on yogurt in order to purchase pure yogurt. Many dairies have sweetened it to make it more popular and have also added:

> modified starch
> corn syrup
> artificial flavor and color
> gelatin
> citric and tartaric acid
> potassium sorbate
> sodium caseinate

none of which are used in making real yogurt. The following are brands which do not have additives: Continental, Yami, Lacto, Colombo, and Dannon, and there may be others. You will find them in the health food stores if not in the supermarket. The Alta-Dena Dairies in California, Continental, and perhaps others produce kefir, a cultured, yogurt-type beverage which can be purchased plain or with fruit flavoring and makes a superb drink. There is also kefir cheese, a delicious, smooth, creamy cheese.

When marketing for eggs, buy fertile eggs, if possible, for

they are more nutritious. Beatrice Trum Hunter tells us that fertile eggs have hormones and vitamin E, that unfertile ones do not, and that some people who are allergic to eggs can tolerate organically raised fertile eggs. It is not known whether the allergy is due to the pesticide residue or chemicals in the feed of the average hens rather than the egg itself, or whether some people can tolerate the fertile egg with its more balanced nutrient content. Also, fertile eggs are fresher because they are locally produced and have a ready turnover. We never know what the age is of the sterile eggs in the supermarket.

Vegetable Oils

In marketing for oils, buy one or several of the nutritious oils: safflower, sunflower, corn, sesame, soybean, peanut, and others or a combination of these. Buy them "pressed," "crude," or "unrefined" in preference to "coldpressed," which term, according to Beatrice Trum Hunter, is meaningless. She says that the source material is heated and partially cooked. Also enormous pressure is exerted to extract the oil which brings additional heat to the process. Yet, it is called "coldpressed." Mrs. Hunter says that if we buy unrefined, pressed oils there is no need for artificial preservatives to be added, since the crude oil contains natural antioxidants such as carotenoids, vitamin E, and phosphatides, all of which help to keep the oil fresh. Vegetable oils lend their own interesting flavors and are excellent for use in salad dressings, seasonings, and for cooking over low heat. Vegetable oils, as noted earlier, are unsaturated fats and contain the essential fatty acids important to good health.

Marketing for real food should become easier not only because health food stores are mushrooming up around us, but because some other markets are making an effort to carry a few of the foods the nutritiously minded will buy. The supermarkets I have seen mark these shelves "Health Foods." We can hope that more grocers will want to make truly natural foods and pure food products available to us.

Chapter 19

General Cooking Methods

Meat, Fish, Fowl

There are two important safeguards to observe when cooking meat. The first is to buy an oven thermometer and be sure your oven temperature is accurate. Otherwise have your oven calibrated. The second safeguard is to cook meat at low temperatures. When meat is cooked at high temperatures, it shrivels and becomes dry and tough. The juices and some of the nutritive value are lost. Do not salt meat before or during cooking; it draws out the juices.

Broil: Brush with oil and broil about five inches from the source of heat unless there is a flame which can be turned down. In that case have the meat about two inches from the flame. I often broil meats and fish with fresh fruits in season. If I cannot purchase fresh fruits, I use unsweetened frozen fruits. For example: when broiling chicken, I brush it with oil and place peach or apricot halves around it and brush the fruit with a little honey. When I broil swordfish steak, I brush it with butter and honey and surround it with pineapple chunks.

Roast: Adelle Davis's all-day method (or all-night method if it means turkey the next noon) is the most convenient and the most satisfactory one I have tried. Brush your roast with oil.

Preheat the oven to 300 degrees and roast it for one hour to destroy surface bacteria. Then lower the temperature to 190 degrees and roast for about ten hours longer. To figure roasting time, triple the time shown on a regular chart and add one hour for the first period. Be sure to use a meat thermometer in roasting. It is one of the best investments you can make.

Stoneware or Crock Pot: Place meat in crock pot. It may be placed on a bed of vegetables if desired. Season, add a small amount of liquid, and cook over low heat for a long period. The time will depend upon the amount of heat used. Electric crock pots have an eight- to ten-hour cooking period.

Pressure Cooker: Use exact recommended timing or less. It cooks vegetables in one minute!

Boil: Do not boil meats; simmer them over very low heat. Simmer meats for soup by bringing the liquid to the simmering point gradually.

Stir Fry: This is the Oriental method of cooking meat and vegetables. Their theory is that the food is cooked long enough to destroy undesirable bacteria but not long enough to destroy the nutritive value. Slice meat thin and cut into small pieces; heat oil in skillet or wok (Chinese pot) and stir while cooking. Do not overcook.

As a family, we are especially fond of Oriental and Polynesian cooking. One dinner I make often is Almond Chicken.

Almond Chicken

> 1 cup brown rice (Cook while preparing remaining recipe. It takes 40 minutes to cook. Follow the recipe on the package.)
> 2 cups diced cooked chicken
> 2 tablespoons butter
> ½ pound mushrooms sliced
> 1 cup (6 oz.) peas (petite if available)
> 1 cup (6 oz.) pea pods
> ½ cup water chestnuts sliced
> ¾ cup chicken broth
> ¼ cup green onions sliced
> 1 tablespoon arrowroot
> 1 tablespoon soy sauce (Kikkoman, Tamari, or other imported Japanese soy sauce)
> ¼ cup slivered almonds browned in butter

Melt butter in a large, heavy skillet, then stir fry onions for

2 minutes. Add peas, pea pods, mushrooms with ½ cup of the broth and simmer, stirring for 3 minutes. Stir arrow-root into remaining ¼ cup of broth and soy sauce. Add with chicken and water chestnuts to mixture in skillet and stir until hot and thickened. Sprinkle with the almonds and serve with the brown rice. Serves four.

Pan Broil or *Sauté:* Cook over low temperatures in a good quality oil or butter. Inasmuch as direct heat pulls out the juices, coat meat first with flour, crumbs, wheat germ, paprika, molasses, or sweetened fruit juice to protect it. Fish may be sautéed quickly in butter. When I sauté filet of sole, I do it in butter with a little sherry. When it is cooked, I place it on a warm platter and quickly sauté peach or apricot halves in the same pan and serve them with the sole.

Vegetables, Fruits, and Salads

In preparing vegetables and fruits, wash carefully not long before cooking time, but do not soak. Fruit and root vegetables should be scrubbed well. Unless we know where our fresh produce comes from, we have to wash off more than dirt—residues from pesticides as well as undesirable waxes and dyes. It is often safest to peel what fruits and vegetables we can and sacrifice the extra nutrition of the peel in lieu of eating chemicals which are not naturally compatible with our systems. When washing lettuce, wash well in cold water and either shake or pat dry with a towel. Place in a plastic bag in the vegetable compartment of the refrigerator to keep crisp.

Except for grains, vegetables should be cooked as briefly as possible to retain food value and beautiful coloring. Vegetables which are considered strong are not strong when cooked a very short time. My mother never allowed cabbage to be cooked longer than five to seven minutes. Then it was drained well, tossed with butter, caraway seeds, and a little salt.

Cook vegetables in as little water as possible; leaf vegetables need only the water remaining on their leaves after washing. Vegetables should be crisp and bright in color. Never add soda, and serve immediately. Do not keep vegetables warm for any period of time. One-third of the nutrients is lost in one hour's time on steam tables. As one nutritionist said of food kept hot for hours on a steam table, "You might as well eat the table."

Waterless Cooking: Ideal. Requires a waterless cooker.

Heavy Pan: Use as little water as possible, about a quarter of an inch, bring to a boil, add vegetables, cover tightly, turn down heat, and cook a few minutes until tender but still crisp. Avoid cooking in aluminum; foods tend to pick up aluminum.

Parchment Paper: Tie vegetables in parchment bag and put into boiling water for required time. Several different vegetables may be cooked at the same time this way.

Steam: Excellent—little loss of nutrients. Steam vegetables on a rack over a small amount of boiling water using the same cooking time as when boiling. Save liquid. Household departments and hardware stores carry steaming racks which can easily be placed in a pot of your own.

Baby's Vegetables: At the time my friends' babies were spitting out their strained, canned beans and spinach, mine were gulping theirs down. The reason? I cooked them according to the above directions for boiling or steaming; then, using a little of the vegetable water (no salt), I whirred them in my blender. I once tasted canned baby food and thought that the babies who spit it out showed good taste; I did not blame them a bit! Besides, they were being robbed of nutrition.

Soups

Soups properly made of natural foods are at the top of the list for aroma, nourishment, and sheer gastronomic delight. Natural food cookbooks abound with intriguing and unique recipes which include the finest meat, fish, and fowl stocks to which have been added vegetable trimmings, all kinds of liquids from the waters in which vegetables and potatoes have been cooked, and liquids in which marvelous things like beans, peas, seeds, and grains have been soaked before sprouting. They also include rich juices from various meats. Furthermore, the recipes call for a wide variety of bean, whole-grain flours, seeds, and every conceivable kind of vegetable, to say nothing of brown rice, whole wheat or artichoke flour noodles, buckwheat dumplings, yogurt, kelp, eggs, fresh lemons, sea salt, and other tantalizing foods.

Stocks are made carefully from meats, fish, or fowl and bones started in cold water and gradually brought to a simmer—

not a boil. Often herbs and carrot, onion, celery, or other stalks are added. The soup is simmered three or four hours (or eight to ten hours in an electric crock pot) and then defatted (either by straining through fine cheesecloth or by placing in the refrigerator so the fat will surface). If a concentrated broth is desired, it is boiled down, uncovered, for a few minutes.

I pour any leftover broth into ice cube trays and freeze. When frozen, I drop the cubes into refrigerator bags. In this way I always have stock on hand. I pull out one or more cubes, dissolve them in a pan over a little heat, and add them to all sorts of sauces and dishes. Below are a few of our family soups.

Consommés

My mother used two special recipes for us when we were sick or recuperating. However, they are elegant soups and appropriate for many occasions. The recipes ordinarily call for regular consommé and can be made with the canned variety if you can find one without sugar or additives.

Consommé Xavier

2 tablespoons milk
1 egg
Pinch of salt and chervil (or other herb)
4 tablespoons whole-wheat pastry flour
1 quart beef tea (recipe below), hot

Beat milk, egg, and salt together; gradually stir in flour and herb. Pour through a strainer into the hot beef tea and simmer a few minutes, stirring briskly with a wire whip. Pour immediately into cups and garnish each with a little piece of parsley or watercress. Serves four.

Consommé Aux Oeufs Pochés

Beef tea (recipe on page 158)
Eggs
Chopped parsley

To each cup of simmering beef tea slip in 1 raw egg and poach it gently. Drain the egg, slip into a cup, pour the beef tea over and sprinkle with chopped parsley.

Or, the hot beef tea can be poured into a warmed cup, the egg slipped into the cup, stirred, and served immediately.

Beef Tea

1 lb. flank steak or 1 lb. lean beef ground
Cold water (spring, preferably), at least 1 cup
½ teaspoon sea salt

Put meat into a quart jar and fill with enough water to cover top of the meat. Add sea salt. Place a dish cloth in the bottom of a deep pan, place the jar on the cloth, fill the pan with as much water as the pan will take without upsetting the jar. Bring to a boil gradually and simmer gently for one hour. Strain into another jar and refrigerate. When ready to use, remove any fat which may have risen to the top. Makes about two cups.

My Cold Avocado Soup

2 medium, ripe avocados
1 cup chicken broth
1 cup half milk-half cream or yogurt
1 tablespoon minced onion
1 teaspoon sea salt

Put all ingredients in a blender and blend well. Chill and serve in soup cups. Garnish with very thin lemon slices cut in half, or nasturtium petals (which are edible).

This soup can be thinned out to a desired consistency with vegetable oil and used as a salad dressing. Serves four or five.

Chapter 20

Excellent Nutritional Foods

For those who are not acquainted with some of the special foods which are high in nutritional value and which can easily be incorporated into daily cooking, I have made a few notations. I will give a brief description of the foods and then a few suggestions for their use.

BREWER'S YEAST (also known as "nutritional yeast" and "primary yeast")

Our cheapest source of vitamin B and our cheapest complete protein, brewer's yeast contains not only a great deal from the vitamin B complex family, but also sixteen amino acids found in protein and 18 minerals. It is low in calories, contains almost no fat, and comes in powdered form.

How to use it: You may have to acquire a taste for brewer's yeast. Experiment to find how it is most palatable for you. Begin with a small amount at first—a half-teaspoonful to a full teaspoonful a day until you are used to it; then increase it gradually up to one or two tablespoons a day, or more if desired.

It can be added to milk, fruit juices, soups, gravies, stews, or meat loaves. It may be mixed with peanut butter and included in whole-grain products. It lends itself to dishes which have strong flavors themselves or when extra spices or herbs with strong aromas are incorporated.

Powdered Nonfat Milk

Some nutritionists feel that powdered nonfat milk is the next best thing to certified raw milk which is more difficult to obtain but the finest milk nutritionally. Get the non-instant which is available in health food stores—the instant kind has gone through more processing and therefore has been robbed of more nutrients.

How to use it: It may be added to liquids and soups and may be used in baking.

Lecithin

Lecithin is found in and is necessary to every cell and organ in the body. Originally lecithin was extracted from egg yolk (which in Greek is "lekithos") but now is made mostly from soybeans.

Lecithin has been found to reduce the cholesterol level in the blood. Egg yolk is a rich source of cholesterol—the rich lecithin content emulsifies the cholesterol. When oils are refined and hydrogenated (as the practice is today), the lecithin in them, tragically enough, is discarded. (For this reason, read labels and avoid hydrogenated foods.)

Lecithin is an excellent source of cholin and inositol; both are B vitamins and necessary to good health. Lecithin also rebuilds cells and tissues in time.

Lecithin may be obtained in capsule, powder, or granule form.

How to use it: From one to four tablespoons of lecithin granules are recommended daily and can be sprinkled on cereals, fruits, salads, yogurt, or stirred into juices.

Soybean Products

Soybeans and products made from soybeans such as soy flour, soy grits, soy flakes, soy oil, and soy milk are an excellent source of vegetable protein. "The carbohydrate content of soybeans is low, and they are especially rich in calcium, phosphorus, and iron; this applies not only to the beans but to the soy flour and grits as well. The green beans contain vitamin A, the B vitamins, and some C. The dry beans have no C and less A but almost three times as much B. The oil has vitamins A and D and is a good source of vitamins E, "F," and K. Vitamin "F" is really a group of special fat constituents known as unsaturated fatty acids. Another virtue of the soybean is that it is rich in lecithin, which is known to be an important component of the sheath around the brain and nerve cells and is also important for the proper functioning of all living cells in the body." [1]

How to use them:

Green Soybeans may be removed from their pods and cooked like lima beans or peas and used as a green vegetable. They can be used in salads, casseroles, fritters. They also come canned or frozen.

Dry Soybeans may be soaked overnight and cooked like lentils with a meaty bone. They may be served with tomato sauce or baked with onions, tomatoes, and other desired ingredients in a casserole or loaf.

Roasted Soybeans (salted) may be used like any salted nut. They are delicious eaten plain or tossed on cereals, salads, broiled fish, and omelets. If preferred, they may be ground first and kept in a tightly sealed jar.

Bean Sprouts may be purchased fresh or canned and may be used raw in salads, cole slaw, and omelets or may be cooked very briefly and used as a vegetable. They may be added to chop suey, chow mein, sukiyaki, egg foo yung, and mixed with other Chinese vegetables.

Soy Grits are quick-cooking and may be cooked as a cereal (1 cup grits to 2 cups water and ½ teaspoon salt—boil 5 minutes) or may be added to vegetable casseroles, meat loaves, hash, croquettes, and soup. For pancakes: 1 cup grits, 1 cup buttermilk, 2 eggs, and ½ teaspoon salt.

Soybean Flour may be added to whole-wheat flour in baking. At Cornell University it was found that a combination of five parts soy flour to ninety-five parts wheat flour not only contained 19% more useable protein than wheat flour alone, but had twice its growth-promoting value. Sesame seeds make an excellent nutritional complement to soy flour and can be used in or on baked goods.

Soy Milk is so palatable and of such high nutritional value that it makes a good beverage. It is available in health food stores. The most nutritious kind is made of dry beans: soak, grind, boil, and take off the water—in other words, the "water extraction method" as compared to the compounded formula. It may be used in all kinds of milk drinks, milk shakes, eggnogs, and in all cooking.

There are hundreds of soybean recipes available in various books.

Yogurt

Yogurt's special values for therapeutic purposes are extensive. It is valuable in offsetting frequent side effects of antibiotic therapy, and is found beneficial in restoring the normal flora of the intestines and at the same time inhibiting undesirable organisms. Yogurt also aids digestion and is beneficial in relieving constipation. The acidity of yogurt increases with storage, and the acid content helps calcium to be assimilated better. It also aids the body's own manufacture of the B vitamins and supplies it with predigested protein. Dr. Cheraskin informs us that

> The cultured milk product (such as yogurt and buttermilk) aids in the digestion and absorption of essential nutrients, by counteracting the discomfort suffered by those older people who lack the enzyme lactase and therefore cannot digest sweet milk. In addition, the microorganisms that ferment milk into buttermilk and yogurt continue their activity in the intestinal tract and actually contribute to the body's manufacture of essential vitamins.[2]

Yogurt has been used since biblical times as a healthful food. To derive the most benefit from it, eat it daily.

How to use: Yogurt may be grown at home or purchased in any grocery store (check to see that there are no additives) or health food store. Add fruit or fruit juices for a pleasant dessert and sprinkle it with nutmeg and/or ground cinnamon if you wish. Yogurt may be used instead of sour cream in recipes.

There are several good books on yogurt-making which include many recipes. Yogurt may be used very satisfactorily in salad dressing, such as the following:

Yogurt Salad Dressing

1 cup yogurt
½ cup vegetable oil
½ cup apple cider vinegar

Combine well and use with salad greens and vegetables. For fruit salad, add a few drops of honey and 1 teaspoon of either celery seeds or poppy seeds.

Carob Powder

The carob plant, like other ancient foods so highly revered in foreign lands, is meeting the needs of Americans today in an exciting way. A powder, which is manufactured from the pods of the carob plant, has the enticement of chocolate but offers extra dividends: more protein, less fat, less carbohydrates, and fewer calories. It is a properly balanced alkaline food which is readily digestible. Carob powder does have a high sugar content, the total sugars being 46.25%, which fact should be taken into consideration by those on sugar-free diets.

The carob tree originates along the shores of the Mediterranean and the Near East. Many names have been given to the carob plant through the years, and these names hold a story in themselves. For example, the most popular name is "St. John's bread," for it is believed that this food sustained John the Baptist during his days in the wilderness; the pods of the carob were called "husks" in the biblical account of the prodigal son; Mohammed's conquering armies existed on these pods and called them "kharub"; the Israelites used the name "boeskur" or "God's bread"; the Romans referred to the food as "carobi" or "bread from the tree"; and the British refer to carob as "honey locust." The carob tree is living up to its noble heritage today in meeting new needs, not the least of which is in bringing a nutritious and delectable food to the modern home.

Carob powder is available in natural food stores across the country and at some supermarkets. You may adapt it to your chocolate recipes by substituting 3 level tablespoons of carob powder plus 2 tablespoons of water per 1 square of chocolate. Carob powder may be successfully used in desired amounts in pancakes, waffles, milk shakes, and baked goods. When our children were growing up, carob brownies were their special treat.

Peanut Butter and Other Nut Butters

Peanut butter is a nutritious food. Use the pure form, non-hydrogenated. Only in recent years has peanut butter been properly labeled. We owe this to the efforts of Mrs. Gordon Desmond, President of the Federation of Homemakers, who is known as the Peanut Butter Grandma, which title she won when the Supreme Court put a final stamp of approval on her eleven-year struggle with the peanut butter makers. She and her lawyers were arrayed against the most highly skilled lawyers in this country, representing such giants in the food industry as Swift, Corn Products, and Proctor and Gamble who make 95% of the peanut butter on the market.

You think you are sending your darling to school with a wholesome peanut butter sandwich; what you are doing, if you use, for example, Proctor and Gamble's "Jif" peanut butter, is sending him to school with a sandwich filled with 22% Crisco— or "peanut flavored cold cream" as Mrs. Desmond describes it. Now you know why it is so easy to spread!

What the chemists and promoters went to work on was a peanut butter to which they added emulsifiers to keep the oil mixed throughout; then they added some sugar to make it sweet to please the sugar-oriented palate industry has created; finally they added hydrogenated (another essentials-robbing process) oil to make it spread easily. Mrs. Desmond contended that if the industry wished to put out a product with less than 90% peanuts in it they should call it "peanut-flavored cream" or some such thing. She won the case; so now when you see a jar of peanut butter, it has to be at least 90% peanuts. However, the 100% peanut butter is still the best and can be obtained in health food stores or stores which have their own nut grinders and make a smooth, pure peanut butter for you while you wait. Nuts and nut butters should be included in the diet. They have good protein value and contain both vitamins and minerals.

Seeds and Sprouting Seeds

We are told by Dr. Bernard Jensen that seeds are some of the most living foods known to man and are thus among the most perfect. Seeds contain nearly every food element discovered and undoubtedly many additional benefits not identified. Jensen says that no other one food is so rich in nutrients as the seed and that from the dawn of time seeds were regarded as life itself. He says that "seeds are nature's vehicle of perpetuity. Tucked away in every kind of seed is the secret of life. Life begets life. Life sustains life."[3] If a seed will sprout, it is alive; both seeds and sprouts, therefore, are valuable foods. Happily for us, they are delicious. The seeds most often used are sunflower, pumpkin, and sesame. They have protein value and, among other nutrients, they contain calcium, phosphorous, iron, vitamins A, B_1 (thiamine), B_2 (riboflavin), B_3 (niacin), D, and E. Sunflower and pumpkin seeds also contain valuable properties in lecithin and the three unsaturated fatty acids (linoleic, linolenic, and arachidonic). These seeds may be obtained raw, roasted, hulled, salted, and unsalted.

How to use seeds: Seeds may be used whole or ground in a blender. They are not only delicious to eat between meals, but are good tossed in salads, sprinkled over soups, fruits, vegetables, and added to yogurt. I like to sprinkle browned sesame seeds on eggs and on an avocado half over the safflower oil and lemon juice I have dropped into its cavity.

How to use sprouts: Sprouts may be used in salads, sandwiches, baked goods, and casseroles or cooked two or three minutes and served as a vegetable. They are easily grown at home, indoors, without soil; they grow within three to five days. Seeds and instructions are available in many health food stores and garden supply houses. Some grown sprouts are available at health food stores and some supermarkets; these are usually bean sprouts and alfalfa sprouts.

Herbs are flowers, leaves, fruits, seeds, roots, barks, and moss, and their basic quality is high. Almost nowhere in the world are they artificially sprayed or fertilized. Herbs lend enchantment to hundreds of foods and are intrinsic to some of the world's most famous dishes. Experimenting with herbs is an adventure.

Herb teas deserve our attention. They are aromatic, fascinating, often mysterious, and always a healthful substitute for coffee or the usual Asian teas and chocolate with their caffeine and theobromine stimulants. A large variety of herb teas are available in most health food stores. The teas are made both of single herbs and in intriguing blends of herbs such as: rose hips, lemon grass, peppermint, spearmint, raspberry leaves, chamomile flowers, eucalyptus, anise, hibiscus flowers, red clover, strawberry leaves, alfalfa, linden leaves, papaya, sage leaves, peach leaves, and many others. Some of these herbs are grown in the United States and others are imported from Bulgaria, Germany, Belgium, Italy, Ireland, and other parts of the world. As a family, we are fond of herb tea. We even use tea in cooking. For instance, sage tea is made of little pieces of sage; it is not crushed nearly as fine as sage prepared for use in cooking. Bob sprinkles his pot roasts with sage tea with very tasty results.

Kelp and dulse are also used as seasonings. They are seaweeds which are rich in vitamins, minerals, and trace elements. They come in powder form to be used as seasoning and in tablet form to be taken as a supplement. Children in Nova Scotia eat dulse like candy.

With such a wide variety of nutritious foods, beautiful seasonings, and types of preparation, we should have no trouble making our family meals attractive. We have only to plan balanced meals with the right foods; such meals are highly satisfying. We must plan good breakfasts of fruit, whole-grain breads or cereals, eggs, and/or meat and well-balanced lunches and dinners which provide high quality protein such as meat, fish, poultry, eggs or cheese, vegetables, crisp salads, properly cooked, nutritious grains, and wholesome desserts. We must not forget to use the same wisdom in our snacks—making them nutritious so they will satisfy and contribute to our well-being. And we must present it all attractively which, by the way, makes it far more interesting to prepare.

Finally, when speaking of health, it would be wrong to leave out two important ingredients: the proper amount of exercise and rest. I have heard nutritionists say that proper exercise and proper rest make proper nutrition work right.

There are many helpful books available on nutrition and marketing nutritiously, and more appear every year. At the back of this book you will find a suggested reading list that will help you in your search for further information.

Chapter 21

Vitamins

It is significant and beautiful that God "never left himself without a witness; there were always his reminders—the kind things he did such as sending you rain and good crops and giving you food and gladness" (Acts 14:17, *Living Bible*). God gave us food as a witness of Himself, and we are stewards of it. But man has removed the vital nutrients God intended for us. Therefore, unless, or until, we can eat the complete foods He provided to fill our hearts with gladness, we can at least supplement them as well as possible. This involves making use of the available knowledge on the vitamins and minerals needed to make up, in so far as we can, for the lack in our daily diet and for whatever individual deficiencies we may have developed or inherited through several generations of eating incomplete and adulterated foods.

Anyone who thinks the average diet supplies all the nutrients we need is living in a dream world. It would seem that even the slightest knowledge of the vitamin and mineral loss in milling, overprocessing, overcooking, and pollution would make it obvious that dietary supplementation is vital to good health today, but it is not yet being widely taught. Hence, many people in the field of health are making statements which were valid in this country over one hundred years ago—but not today. Anthropologist Ernest Hooton of Harvard succinctly expressed such oversight of the obvious when he said, "Really gifted scientists are those who can appreciate the obvious." The simple is hard to accept.

Vitamin E

The vitamin most under attack, I believe, is vitamin E. Some medical traditionalists have erected a barrier against it, although it is being widely used in England, Germany, France, Italy, and Russia. Monumental work on vitamin E has been done by Dr. Wilfred Shute and his brother in Canada and many others elsewhere. Shute has written two important books on vitamin E, *Vitamin E for Ailing and Healthy Hearts* (with Harold J. Taub) and *Complete-Updated Vitamin E Book.* These books come out of many years of research and experience with vitamin E.

The interesting point that Shute makes, after his thirty-six years of practice and the more than thirty thousand patients whom he has been called upon to treat or to supervise in treatment, is that the lack of vitamin E in our daily diet is a direct factor in heart disease. "Today we know that the natural antithrombin in the bloodstream is a chemical called alpha tocopherol. . . . alpha tocopherol is one of a group of compounds . . . which collectively are known as vitamin E. It is an oil-soluble vitamin which is stored in the fatty tissues of the body." [1] In 1870 the high-speed roller was invented which eliminated the essential nutrient, vitamin E, the antithrombin, from flour. In 1900 coronary disease was unknown. Today, with the further refining of grains and oils, heart disease is our biggest killer. Shute maintains that this need not be the case.

Shute goes into detail in his books about the successful and well-documented results obtained from the use of vitamin E in connection with other problems. At a meeting of the International Academy of Preventive Medicine, I saw the most unbelievable pictures taken by the Shute Foundation of the "before and after" in cases of bad burns treated with vitamin E; the burns were completely healed and there was no contraction of scar tissue. Ever since seeing this demonstration, I have used vitamin E in my home, and it is the most effective first-aid remedy for burns I have ever used. There is always a vitamin

E capsule in my kitchen. The instant a burn occurs, I pierce the capsule, squeeze the liquid onto the burn, and place a Band-Aid over it. I have never had such instant relief nor rapid healing of minor burns, and I recommend the remedy.

To be noted, however, is a word of caution in regarding the use of vitamin E ointment. Dr. Shute warns: "About 10% of people cannot tolerate the full strength ointment on open wounds or ulcers. Before being applied to the whole area, vitamin E should always be used on one corner of the ulcer or sore until it is evident that it does not cause a local reaction.... The ointment is a 30 International Unit per gram of alpha tocopherol in a petroleum jelly base." [2] Either a half-strength dilution may benefit without reaction or the powder from a capsule of succinate.

Uninformed sources say vitamin E is found in so many foods that it is almost impossible for humans to develop a vitamin E deficiency. However, laboratories in the United States and in Europe show the loss of vitamin E in food processing to be great. According to Shute, 87% of vitamin E is lost in milling by removing the germ from wheat; the remainder is successfully removed in the bleaching process. He says, "The alpha tocopherol (vitamin E) content of whole maize, wheat, oats and rice goes down by as much as 90% when they are made into breakfast cereals.... Vitamin E has also been almost completely removed from refined hydrogenated oils, soy and cottonseed margarines, mayonnaise and other items of this kind." [3]

Doctors experienced in vitamin therapy, biochemists, and nutritionists all tell us that vitamin E plays a role as a protection against damage to the lungs from pollution. We are also told that the more polyunsaturates we consume, the greater our need for vitamin E. Shute says that "if a physician prescribes a diet rich in polyunsaturated fats, he is dropping the already marked deficiency of vitamin E way below critical level. If you consume such a diet, it reduces the antithrombin in your bloodstream and thus encourages, produces or precipitates clots in blood vessels." [4]

Most people seem to take from 400 to 800 international units of vitamin E daily. The recommended dose may be twice that in some cases. It is important, however, that people with high blood pressure are not given even 400 IUs to start with; a considerably lower dose is recommended and should be prescribed by a professional in the field of vitamin therapy.

Dr. Harold Rosenberg states: "It is possible that vitamin E deficiencies or low-reserve states could exist for a decade or longer without being noticed. The effects on general circulation and overall physical strength resulting from such a long-term deficiency could be profound, even for those who do not have heart attacks or strokes owing to blood clots." [5]

Contrary to common belief, a great deal of research on vitamin E is in progress, and great strides are being made. Hardly a month goes by that we do not hear of doctors discovering for themselves some benefit from the use of vitamin E.

Vitamin C

Vitamin C, like E, has been the cause of much controversy. No vitamin, however, has had more thorough research done on it over a longer period of years by extremely capable scientists, both here and in various parts of the world, than vitamin C. Dr. Linus Pauling, our most eminent authority on the subject, vouches for the efficiency of vitamin C in many areas. His important book is *Vitamin C and the Common Cold.* Drs. Harold Rosenberg and A. N. Feldzamen inform us, in their book *The Doctor's Book of Vitamin Therapy,* of these findings:

It has long been known that a prolonged lack of vitamin C produces the mortal disease of scurvy—and lesser insufficiencies often lead to bleeding gums, blood vessel fragility (producing many black-and-blue marks on the skin), bone and teeth weakness in growing children, anemia, general debility, and an increased susceptibility to infections.

The latest research verifies that vitamin C in large amounts does protect us against colds and minor illnesses, promotes the healing of wounds and injuries, and may also sharpen mental abilities.

Soldiers under the extreme stress and tension of battlefield combat have drastically reduced vitamin C reserves in their bodies, indicating this vitamin has important anti-stress properties.

In addition this vitamin aids in the absorption of iron into the body, helps overcome foreign poisons, has been useful in treating schizophrenia and ulcers, has helped cataract patients. . . .

Vitamin C is used in every living cell in the fundamental metabolic processes of life and also has special functions in the white blood cells (which fight infection) and in the manufacture of collagen, a binding substance that holds all cells and the bones together. Further, there is growing evidence that vitamin C protects the circulatory system against damaging fatty deposits.[6]

Dr. Rosenberg tells us that vitamin C deficiency is likely to cause high cholesterol levels. Of special significance to almost everyone in these days is that "Vitamin C often prevents or counteracts poisonings from such toxic agents as the metals lead, arsenic, and other poisons such as carbon monoxide, benzines, bromides and severe overdoses of aspirin. Insect bites, as well as poison ivy and poison oak, can also be detoxified by vitamin C."[7]

We have learned that vitamins E and A help protect us from pollution; it is important to know that vitamin C is also effective in overcoming air, water, and food pollution. Again we see the vital role vitamin supplementation plays in our health today. We are not only eating depleted foods, but most of us have to fight pollution of one kind or another.

We do hear from uninformed sources that tests have been run on vitamin C which prove its inefficacy. It is said that one group of people was given vitamin C while another received placebos. Those with vitamin C fared no better. We do not hear, however, how much vitamin C was given nor for what period of time, and herein lies the fault with many tests that are made. I have heard a number of experts in megavitamin therapy, including Pauling and Shute, say that tests for vitamin therapy are often not given properly: too little of the vitamin over too short a period of time has been given in the unfavorable tests they have uncovered. A doctor would be the first to tell you that a fraction of his prescribed drug over too short a period would not do the job, but many doctors will not use the same logic in administering vitamins therapeutically. We may also note that our systems do not have to recover from doses of vitamins as they do from drugs which are an assault on the system. And I have been told by doctors experienced in vitamin therapy that although in rare cases large doses of vitamins produce adverse reactions, the symptoms disappear as soon as the vitamins are stopped.

I certainly see this in my friends. I have watched many take from 100 to 500 milligrams of vitamin C daily to ward off a cold with no success. It would be impossible to tell anyone how many colds I have thwarted by taking vitamin C at the onset— but I take from 8,000 to 10,000 milligrams a day: 2,000 four times a day. For infection, 1,000 to 2,000 milligrams an hour are often very effective. Doctors experienced in the field administer many times that amount by injection for therapeutic results.

Some persons feel they cannot tolerate vitamin C in large doses, and Pauling says that this is sometimes a problem. He believes a person is not allergic to synthetic vitamin C but, rather, to its excipients (the substance which forms the vehicle for the vitamin). He adds that the rose hips (vitamin C in a natural form) preparations have changed; in many cases the vitamin used is synthetic with a little rose hips added (pure rose hips, one may note, is very brown). Pauling believes that the pure crystalline C is safest where excipients present a problem.

Lesser-Known Vitamins

Dr. Armand J. Quick, a researcher on the staff of the Medical College of Wisconsin, reports a vitamin Q in soybeans. Linda Clark, in her book *Know Your Nutrition,* describes two B vitamins we do not hear about. They are B_{15} and B_{17} which she says have been condemned in the U.S., not because they are dangerous—actually they are nontoxic—but because the government insists there is no evidence of proof that they are helpful.[8]

Some researchers have found these vitamins of value. Pangamic acid, B_{15}, Miss Clark says, is considered a life-saving vitamin in Russia. They have found it helpful in certain heart conditions and in the early healing of muscles of injured legs. They also find that it improves physical energy, and they combine it with vitamins A and E in a product they call Aevit which they claim is very effective. Germany offers four or five ethical brands of B_{15}, Miss Clark tells us and, interestingly enough, the vitamin was originally isolated here in the States by Dr. Ernst T. Krebs and his son of San Francisco.[9] Dr. Cheraskin writes that

Dr. Alan Cott, a pioneer researcher in megavitamin therapy for disturbed children, includes vitamin B_{15} in his treatment for hyperactive children and for children with learning disabilities and has successfully used B_{15} in youthful schizophrenia. Cott has traveled to Russia to study their vitamin programs. The Russians have found dosages of B_{15} promising in their treatment of mental retardation. Cheraskin adds that B_{15} has not yet been seriously investigated in the United States, but Soviet scientists believe that it aids in the respiration of brain tissue.[10]

Also, according to Linda Clark, B_{17}, the medical dosage forms of which are known as Laetrile and Amygdalin, is made in Mexico where they believe it is helpful for some forms of cancer. This caused 2,500 of our cancer sufferers who could not get help here to go to Mexico, and much controversy ensued. The controversy still rages with apparently about 5,000 persons in the U.S. claiming benefits from Laetrile and some doctors and researchers claiming positive evidence of therapeutic value in testing mice.[15] Still, other well-known foundations contradict these claims because they did not get the same results in their tests. The FDA does not see sufficient reason to run tests on humans, but we may be hearing more about Laetrile in years hence. E. T. Krebs says the diet of primitive man was very high in B_{17}, and we can get it in whole natural foods.

There is a difference in nonbiological drugs and the natural nutrients that are needed by the cells in our bodies. One of the greatest mysteries of the twentieth century is why the natural takes so long to be accepted. Many of us have had doctors prescribe medicines for us, which are foreign to our body chemistry, without the blink of an eyelid; but the same doctors are skeptical, even negative, about these vitamins which God provides in the food we eat!

There is a difference between natural and synthetic vitamins, some of which can make a difference, and this should be understood. There is constant controversy over it. The actual vitamin per vitamin in the natural and synthetic is the same and has to be so labeled. The reason that some nutritionists prefer the natural over the synthetic is because of the possible elements not yet identified in the natural which they feel could, and probably do, make a difference in many cases. In other words, natural vitamins, from fresh food, come together with naturally related food factors. We know that vitamins and minerals work together. Science does not know all of the associated food factors which are necessary in human nutrition. Nature does. However, the efficacy of the synthetic product, especially used therapeutically in megavitamin (massive) doses cannot be overlooked.

The one-a-day variety of good quality vitamin-mineral supplement is fine if the ingredients are complete enough and in sufficient potency. Most of us, however, need further supplementation. We can start out with deficiencies—many mothers were not properly nourished during pregnancy, the soil some of our food has come from has been deficient—and we create deficiencies as we go along. For instance, according to Pauling, smoking and air pollution destroy vitamin C; this is on top of the deficiencies caused by our other bad habits and poor diet. If we had always eaten well of vegetables grown in good soil and animals fed properly, if we had always avoided overprocessed foods, refined bread and cereal, and sugar, if we had always had good living habits and breathed clean air, we would not need supplements.

RDA (Recommended Daily Allowance)

The food products which contain vitamin and mineral additives list them in accordance with the U.S. RDA (Recommended Daily Allowance as the "official measurement of nutritional intake" to quote the FDA). The RDA replaces the MDR (Minimum Daily Requirement) designation formerly used. Neither term is useful according to the respected vitamin experts of our country. As one senator wrote me: "The FDA regulations are based upon a system of arbitrarily designated recommended daily allowances. A federal court has found that no scientific basis has been demonstrated by the FDA for the establishment of such allowances and many eminent scientists have questioned them." The most the RDA can mean, perhaps, is that it is the minimum amount needed to protect one from acute stages of malnutrition. It hardly refers to amounts known to contribute to health. Also, "Dr. Linus Pauling, Dr. Leon Rosenberg, Dr. Abram Hoffer and Dr. Humphrey Osmond have indicated that fixed levels of vitamins, as noted by the RDA, 'fail to achieve cellular balance.' " [11]

Senator William Proxmire says that the RDA is based on an "arbitrary, unscientific and tainted standard." He explains that the FDA standard is established by the Food and Nutrition Board of the National Research Council which is influenced, dominated, and financed in part by the food industry. He says that it represents one of the most scandalous conflicts of interest in the federal government. As an example, Senator Proxmire cites the fact that the chairman of the Food and Nutrition Board, who occupies an academic chair funded by the Mead-Johnson baby food company, appeared at the FDA vitamin hearings not only as an FDA-government witness but also on behalf of such firms as Mead-Johnson and Abbott Laboratories. Senator Proxmire says that the Food and Nutrition Board, which establishes the RDA, establishes low RDAs because the lower the RDAs, the more nutritional the products appear that are put out by the food industry which heavily finances the Food and Nutrition Board—hence the "scandalous conflicts of interest." [12]

Recent action taken in Washington concerning vitamins demonstrates not only the growing public awareness for the need of vitamin supplementation, but also the sovereignty of the people in our nation when they are aroused enough to voice their opinions. As most of us know, the FDA was formed to protect us from contaminated food and to prevent the marketing and distribution of danger drugs. In recent years the FDA has wanted to legislate on vitamins—a move many outraged citizens feel far exceeds their authority.

The FDA decreed that any vitamin containing more than 150% of the Recommended Daily Allowance (their completely arbitrary and extremely low figure) must be sold as a drug. This meant two things: First, vitamins they considered harmless would be sold in such small potencies that users, in many cases, would have to buy many tablets instead of one to attain the portion they knew best for their health. For instance, those taking 1000 milligrams of vitamin C (not an uncommon daily dose) would have to buy and daily swallow eleven tablets instead of one or two. To ward off a cold, I would have to buy and swallow ninety tablets a day instead of three.

Secondly, the vitamins that FDA considers potentially harmful, A and D, would have to be prescribed by doctors in a potency higher than 10,000 IU (International Units). It so happens that 10,000 IU is less than one-third the amount of vitamin A found in two ounces of liver or a half cup of cooked spinach. As far as vitamin D is concerned, Senator Proxmire tells us about an absurdity of the FDA rulings on this vitamin: It seems that while on one hand they are saying that 400 IU is potentially dangerous, on the other hand they are requiring that a quart of milk contain the equivalent of 1,200 to 4,000 IU of vitamin D! There is no disputing the fact that vitamin A and D can be harmful if taken in colossal doses over a long period of time; it is the unreasonably low, the ineffectually low potency the FDA wishes to impose which is the issue.

Constructive Voices in Washington

We have had strong voices of protest in Washington; Senator Proxmire introduced an important bill to block the FDA ruling, and it passed! He says in no uncertain terms that the FDA "in their zeal and hostility has thrown up a group of strawmen, distorted statements, and outright misstatements of fact and scientific evidence. They are myth makers." [13] Senator Proxmire further states that the FDA has been turning out propaganda for years in their attempt to smear the entire health food movement. In order to win their battle, Senator Proxmire contends they have thrown out a smokescreen to cover up their intentions.

We do have congressmen in Washington who are realistic in their views of what is needed for the nation's health and who are taking definite action. Senators William Proxmire, Richard Schweiker, George McGovern, Edward Kennedy, and Frank Church have been in the forefront. We have diligent groups like the Center for Science in the Public Interest and the Federation of Homemakers who work incessantly to protect the health of the nation. And we have a man like Dr. Miles H. Robinson, who has served as medical advisor on the staffs of two senators during six years of their investigation of the Food and Drug Administration and who gives a great deal of his time and energy protecting our interests in the fields of food and drugs. He has just spent two exhausting years representing the National Health Federation by testifying in the vitamin issues in the U.S. Court of Appeals.

All these people need our support if we want every chance

for good health for ourselves and the generations to come. Our influence can be felt in Washington. It was when so many thousands of citizens wrote to their congressmen protesting the original vitamin rulings the FDA attempted to put into effect that the rulings were held up. Those of us who are interested are going to have to stay with the cause and keep abreast of further developments in Washington. We are called upon to "be vigilant" (1 Peter 5:8); surely this pertains to every area of our lives, including our health.

Legalized Health Hazards

We, as Christian stewards, must be informed. We know this. Furthermore, if we are interested in the health of our nation, we do well to understand the inconsistency between the vitamin rulings the FDA proposed and the allowances made on drugs and cigarettes. For instance, fifty tons of aspirin are consumed daily in the United States. Beyond this, according to pharmacist Milton Silverman and Dr. Philip R. Lee in their book *Pills, Profits & Politics,* there are 30,000 deaths annually due to legal drugs, legally obtained, mostly by prescription, and used only with bona fide medical intentions. The authors say that adverse drug reactions kill more victims than does breast cancer in women, and that 30 to 40% of all hospital patients suffer adverse reactions.[14] If all this goes on, isn't it out of line for the FDA to impose drastic restrictions on healthful food supplements?

Fifty-six million people smoke an average of twenty-seven cigarettes a day. An obvious inconsistency of the FDA, which comes under HEW (the Department of Health, Education and Welfare), is to concern itself with making it obligatory to procure a doctor's prescription for certain potencies of vitamins and not demand that the public obtain a prescription for cigarettes which are *definitely* harmful to everyone. Instead, our government gives more money to subsidize tobacco than to research the destructive effects of tobacco upon us.

In conclusion, we do need good quality vitamin and mineral supplementation, but we must not let even the best supplementation take the place of eating properly. We want all the nutrients we know about and all we don't know about, and we want them in their whole, natural state in our food.

PART 6

Could This Be You?

Dear friend, I pray that you may enjoy good health and that all may go well with you, even as your soul is getting along well.

3 John 2

Chapter 22

Sugar: When More Means Less

The diet of most Americans today, as demonstrated in previous chapters, causes a variety of debilitating physical and mental conditions. One of the most distressing of these conditions is hypoglycemia, or low blood sugar. Because of the number of people who suffer from this condition (at least 20% of our nation, according to doctors working on the problem), and because the condition is overlooked or misdiagnosed by many doctors, I felt it was important to include a chapter on it in this book.

Hypoglycemia may be a problem of yours, of a family member, a friend, or someone you are working with or counseling. Just four years ago, I learned that it is a problem I have inherited and have been living with all my life. Therefore, I write from a lifetime of experience with it and now many months of study, numerous interviews with informed doctors, and attendance at several national medical meetings relating to the subject. I have also investigated carefully all the cases I have come across among my friends and acquaintances. They have responded remarkably to the correct treatment, as I have.

What is Hypoglycemia?

Cases of hypoglycemia can be divided into those which are organic and those which are functional or relative. Organic hypoglycemia is caused by a tumor or other disease of the endocrine glands involved in metabolism; this type is quite rare. Functional hypoglycemia, the type seen more frequently, is the one with which this and the following chapter will deal.

Functional hypoglycemia can be caused by one or more of several conditions: an inherited glandular or biochemical predisposition toward it; chronic stress; temporary but severe stress; insufficient nutrients in the diet or poor absorption of them; consumption of large amounts of alcohol; and consumption of large amounts of carbohydrates—starches and refined sugar. The relationship between hypoglycemia and alcohol will be considered in the following chapter. The effects of diet and refined sugar will be considered here.

As described earlier, one of the most significant differences between the diets of primitive peoples and our own today is the amount of sugar available and consumed. Dr. H. J. Roberts, a director of research in internal medicine, explains this difference clearly and suggests one of the damaging consequences for us today:

(a) The amount of sugar primitive man could eat was strictly limited by the amount of bulk from natural foods his stomach could hold;
(b) when primitive man ate sugar, he also had to eat protein, vitamins, minerals and other food elements along with it, and
(c) his sugar supply came mainly from plant starch, which the body breaks down only gradually into glucose.

In stark contrast, modern man:

(a) gobbles down pound after pound of sugar without being restrained by so much as a thread of fibre;
(b) eats sugar without getting a trace of any vital nutrient (except calories), not even those which are necessary to help metabolize the sugar, and
(c) brutalizes his islets of Langerhans (the section of the pancreas which releases insulin) by eating all the sugar in the form of sucrose, which instead of breaking down into glucose gradually, turns into the critical sugar al-

most immediately. No wonder the cells that must se-
crete insulin to deal with all this sugar go haywire![1]

Dr. Miles H. Robinson describes the process of sucrose
turning into critical sugar almost immediately:

> While sugar does provide quick energy, which may be
> useful in an emergency, it is like burning gasoline in a
> home furnace. It will burn, but it wrecks the machinery.
> (The design of the body resembles not a gas but a diesel
> engine, which is more efficient, and gets its more powerful
> stroke from *a slower burning* of a cruder fuel.)[2]

It has been estimated that in 1750 the average person in
England ate about 4 pounds of sugar per year. In 1850, the
amount was 25 pounds per year. Today, the amount has jumped
to at least 104 pounds each year for each person in both England and the U.S.—and many adults eat far more. In other words,
on an average, we eat our weight in sugar each year! Our bodies
and our endocrine and metabolizing systems were not designed
to cope with such an influx of sugar; many of us simply cannot
accommodate it. When we try, the consequences are destructive
and the symptoms are numerous, varying widely from one
person to another.

Symptoms

A physician in Florida, Dr. Stephen Gyland, was a victim
of rapid pulse, severe headaches, fatigue, arthritis, blurred vi-
sion, and blackouts. He was given tests for a suspected brain
tumor. He went to fourteen specialists and three nationally
known clinics and was finally told by a neurologist that he was
finished for life and would never see another patient. The diagnosis was cerebral arteriosclerosis. Fortunately, his coordinat-
ing doctor had ordered a six-hour glucose tolerance test (the test
which measures blood sugar levels). When the test indicated
low blood sugar, Dr. Gyland went on a four-month search to
find out all he could about hypoglycemia. He turned up Dr.
Seale Harris's work on the subject and began immediately to
follow the recommended diet. Gyland's wife describes the results: "His recovery was like a miracle and was the answer to
fervent prayers."

Because the endocrine system is so intricate, interdependent, and interworking, the symptoms of hypoglycemia are extremely varied, even bizarre. It is the divergence and the number of these symptoms that make some people doubtful about the importance of hypoglycemia, and even about its existence. A frequent comment is that no *one* disorder can cause so many different kinds of problems. The simplest explanation for this was given to me by our doctor, an endocrinologist; he pointed out that "when the glands are off, anything can be off; the system is out of balance."

Dr. Carlton Fredericks reports that after Gyland realized that it had been hypoglycemia which had caused him such distress, he treated over six hundred people who also had hypoglycemia. In the course of their treatment, he recorded the following symptoms:

Nervousness	Mental confusion
Exhaustion	Crying spells
Irritability	Muscle cramps or jerking
Dizziness	Numbness
Fainting spells	Uncoordination
Tremor	Lack of concentration
Weak spells	Indecisiveness
Depression	Unsocial, antisocial behavior
Forgetfulness	Noises in the ears
Digestive disturbances	Allergies
Headaches	Blurred vision
Drowsiness	Gasping for breath
Wakefulness	Smothering spells
Unprovoked anxiety	Yawning, sighing
Chronic worrying	Tingling of lips
Trembling internally	Itching and crawling sensa-
Heart palpitations	tions
Phobias and fears	Neurodermatitis
Nightmares, night terrors	Rheumatoid arthritis
Nervous breakdown	Suicidal intent[3]

Dr. Carlton Fredericks has said that his research reveals that 60% of the psychiatric cases tested in a group outside the hospital and 60% of the patients tested in a mental hospital had hypoglycemia.

Hypoglycemia has important implications for diagnosticians. Its symptoms can imitate those of many health problems, including ulcers and heart attacks. Dr. Demetrio Sodi Pallares, who is chief of the National Heart Institute in Mexico City, says that hypoglycemia will give a false electrocardiogram reading of a heart attack. He reports that research started several months ago shows that many cases diagnosed as disease of the heart actually are disorders of metabolism.

Mental health is certainly one of the most perplexing and debilitating conditions in America today. Dr. William Cole summarizes the conclusions of an important medical investigator:

> Dr. Macmilian Fabrykant, of New York University Medical School, has been studying hypoglycemia for nearly a half century and exhorting his skeptical colleagues to take it as seriously as he and many other physicians do. Dr. Fabrykant believes that inadequate blood sugar is responsible for a great deal of mental illness, the nation's foremost health problem. "When the content of the sugar in the blood declines to abnormal levels," he says, "all tissues except the brain may derive energy from the other main fuel sources —proteins and fat. The brain is dependent almost exclusively upon blood-sugar for food and oxygen, for it cannot absorb and use oxygen without the presence of sugar. Thus, the degree of the sugar shortage, the brain is starved and suffocated. The resulting interference with central nervous system function and metabolism can lead—in severe cases—to permanent brain damage and death." [4]

Of course, there can be other causes for these same symptoms, among them mineral deficiencies and imbalances in body chemistry, and these were touched upon earlier. Also, other physical problems can accompany hypoglycemia, or the cause can be organic (in the form of a tumor, for instance). Therefore, the layman must not jump to the conclusion that he is suffering from functional hypoglycemia or from hypoglycemia alone. A complete check-up by a competent doctor specializing in the field of hypoglycemia is imperative.

I sincerely believe, however, when a person has one or several symptoms mentioned and has already gone to doctors, has had all sorts of tests, and ends up with no satisfactory explanation or help, it would be tragic not to find a doctor who does understand hypoglycemia better. And, in the meantime, someone suspecting hypoglycemia should go on the diet; it is a healthful one, and improvement may be felt in a comparatively short time. I have seen it happen many times.

Tests

Hypoglycemia is sometimes missed because an inadequate test has been made. Often glucose levels are tested for only one to three hours. The experts tell me that this is a test for diabetes and is not adequate in determining hypoglycemia. Blood sugar often does not fall into levels that are too low until the fourth or fifth hours. Whether or not a person has hypoglycemia should therefore be determined only after a five or six hour test.

Furthermore, the longer test is sometimes misinterpreted. Some look to see if the levels remain within the "normal" range. This can be very misleading, however, because the pattern of fluctuation, even within the range is equally important. My sugar levels were within the "normal" range, yet, I am actually hypoglycemic. During the third hour of the test my sugar level drops very sharply; this plays havoc with my system and all my distressing symptoms descend upon me. This is what used to happen to me to some degree every few hours all day long, year after year, and my problem was never suspected.

Wrong Treatment

There is a further problem. Sometimes even if appropriate tests are given and hypoglycemia is accurately diagnosed, a harmful treatment can be prescribed for it, namely sugar. I know of a man who is the father of nine and has hypoglycemia. He has been unable to work steadily for years. His condition was correctly diagnosed as hypoglycemia years ago by doctors. He was told by these doctors to eat candy. Rather than stabilizing his condition, this, of course, aggravated his symptoms. The result is that he has to admit himself to the hospital periodically because of blackouts.

The Undiagnosed

Too many people, even if they are not tormented by prescribed treatment opposite to the one they need, are bearing varying degrees of aggravated symptoms because their conditions are undiagnosed. I know several people who are such wrecks they will not go to the doctor; in fact, they seldom go anywhere. They have seen many doctors and many psychiatrists and all to no avail. Some have had Christian counseling as well. There comes a time when one has told one's story in vain so often that one stops telling it even to doctors and simply withdraws from life. These people often accuse themselves of too little faith, which some friends, like Job's friends, have implied; this only compounds their unexplained misery. These people may not be hypoglycemic; only medical tests and the services of a knowledgeable doctor can determine that for certain. But I do know of many cases like these which have been tested, found hypoglycemic, and treated successfully. This is why I grieve over anyone so badly off who has not at least been tested for the possibility of low blood sugar. And I grieve when I pass mental institutions because I wonder how many people are there who do not belong there at all. A further tragedy is that the diet in most such institutions contributes to the patients' ill health.

The Positive Side

Fortunately, there is an increasing number of doctors who are thoroughly acquainted with hypoglycemia and its related conditions, as well as with the correct tests and treatments for it. There is also an increasing amount of promising research being done in this area. Some doctors, on the basis of their own and others' research, and on the basis of their experience with thousands of cases of hypoglycemia, have now begun to specialize in this area.

Other individuals have taken note: parents, pastors, doctors, psychiatrists, researchers, and anthropologists are among them. Their findings are fascinating, and the practical implications of their findings are critical.

Hypoglycemia in Children

The benefits of early diagnosis and care are far-reaching indeed. Dr. Hugh W. S. Powers, Jr., a pediatrician with over twenty years of experience, has spent the past several years doing work on blood sugar levels. He tested 260 children's sugar levels and found that the nearer the levels are brought to a normal curve (or pattern of fluctuation), the better the performance of the child. He noted that drug users run low blood sugar levels. Among symptoms he found in hypoglycemic children were sullenness and irritability. These children were often called dumb or stupid in school. After treatment for hypoglycemia, he found definite improvement in both their disposition and their achievement. Relapses came when the children went off their diet and back to usual cake, potato chip, candy, soft drink type of diet common to children today.

Others have reported startling results with the treatment of hypoglycemia in youth. There are many cases of changed personalities, accelerated motivation, and healthy, responsive, constructive attitudes. When the condition is not treated, however, the consequences can be serious.

The consequences for the underprivileged children in society can be especially serious. Young people living in poverty usually subsist on very poor diets. Such diets can cause or aggravate hypoglycemia. Hypoglycemia, in turn, has been shown to be related to unsocial and antisocial behavior. Underprivileged people may, therefore, have physiological reasons, as well as emotional and psychological reasons, for engaging in delinquent and criminal activities. There is increasing evidence, in fact, that hypoglycemia is closely related to delinquency and crime.

Similarly, for the past half-century, the diet of even the privileged and overprivileged children in our society, in spite of all its abundance, has been sadly lacking in the vital body-building, endocrine-balancing, brain-sustaining nutrients. Hypoglycemia has, therefore, become more widespread. At the same time that the nation's diet has become more and more deficient and hypoglycemia has increased, the rate of delinquency, crime, alcohol consumption, and drug addiction has also increased.

We must look at all "problem" children in a new light. I am told by doctors who know about the dangers of hypoglycemia that we must listen carefully to the complaints of our children, and we must closely watch their actions. We must notice what they eat and try to see if there is any connection between what they eat, *when* they eat, and how they behave. It is vital, for them and for *their* children, that we understand them, feed them nutritiously, and find for them a competent doctor who is thoroughly familiar with hypoglycemia and nutrition.

Hypoglycemia in Drivers and Pilots

Children, of course, are not the only ones whose performance can be affected by hypoglycemia. The efficient, safe-functioning of adults can also be affected, including those who carry responsibilities for the lives of others—automobile drivers and pilots, for example. Dr. H. J. Roberts, who is also an expert on traffic accidents, explains that a drop in blood sugar levels causes absentmindedness, drowsiness, and blackouts. In other words, hypoglycemia can be, and has been, responsible for many automobile accidents.[5]

Mr. Mark Bricklin provides some details: "In many of these tragedies, the truth is that the driver had one too many—one too many desserts, pieces of candy, slices of cake, or any other sugar-laden processed food." [6] We all know people who take colas, coffee, or other forms of caffeine to keep awake, but we do not stop to think of the decline which follows.

In 1969, Dr. Charles R. Harper made a study of hypoglycemia among 175 pilots over the age of forty. There seemed to be enough evidence of hypoglycemic symptoms among United States pilots to warrant a study on the subject by the Federal Aviation Administration. The result was that forty-four of the pilots tested showed a drop of blood sugar level of some concern, but they had no other symptoms at the time. Two years later, thirty of the forty-four reported such symptoms as drowsiness, irritability, unclear thinking, tremors, faintness, and digestive troubles. They were all put on a hypoglycemia diet; this took care of the problem and none of the pilots had to be grounded.

Contrasting Patterns of Diet and Behavior in Remote Areas

Because of our diet, therefore, and because of the stresses under which we live, many Americans have not been able to enjoy the full potential of their bodies and their personalities.

It is instructive to note, however, that the Hunzakuts, who live high up in the Himalayas and eat all the natural, nutritious foods of the area, exhibit ideal personality characteristics.

Another group, on the other hand, the Qolla, who live

high up in the Andes in Peru, suffer as we do—perhaps even more so. Professor Ralph Bolton, of the Department of Anthropology at Pomona College, lived with the Qolla for five years and gives us a fascinating account of them. Professor Bolton observes: first, the Qolla have a poor diet; this is the result of overpopulation and scarcity of pastures which allows them to raise only a few animals. Their poor diet is also the result of over-utilization and poor fertilization of their soil, causing a depletion of nutrients. Furthermore, their capricious weather ruins their crops year after year. Secondly, the Qolla chew coca (the plant from which coca cola derives an ingredient) and drink excessively; this immediately raises the glucose levels in their blood. Thirdly, the Qolla live under certain environmental and cultural stresses.

The Qolla have been known by several investigators as hostile, distrustful, fearful, self-pitying, submissive, anxious, sullen, apprehensive, emotionally unstable, melancholic, noncommunicative, morose, cruel, quarrelsome, and irrational. Given the environmental and dietary conditions, as well as the emotional instability of the Qolla, it is not surprising that Professor Bolton suspected a high rate of hypoglycemia among them. He gave glucose tolerance tests to sixty-six Qolla men who represented heads of families. The tests showed that fully 55.5% of them appeared to have hypoglycemia.[7] This, then, is one more example of the relationship of nutrition to health and behavioral patterns. And it is encouraging to know that some anthropologists are looking at the biochemical basis of cultural behavior and mental illness.

Diet for Hypoglycemia

In conclusion, may I say that the hypoglycemia diet is a wonderful one. I have been interested in international cooking all my life, have written and lectured on it, and still spend happy hours experimenting with new recipes. I cannot imagine complaining about a diet that provides meat, fish, poultry, vegetables, salads, salad dressings, fruits, nuts, all the dairy products including butter, eggs, and all the marvelous cheeses in the world, as well as the herbs, spices, and seasonings which give unlimited variety and interest to dishes. A good breakfast is important, as well as eating a little something every two to three hours to keep the blood sugar level from dropping. Snacks can be cheese, nuts, fruit, milk, hard-boiled egg, or leftover protein from a meal.

It would seem that eating sugar would be the answer to low blood sugar. The correct treatment, however, is quite the opposite. The worst thing to do is to eat sweets because the blood sugar level then shoots up only to drop sharply to abnormal levels; the pick-up feels fine, but great is the drop thereof! The only way to achieve and maintain the proper balance is to eat the foods which convert slowly into sugar and to eat often. Proteins and fat (meat, poultry, fish, dairy products) convert the most slowly, vegetables next, then fruit. Refined carbohydrates (starches and sugar) convert the most quickly. Consequently, natural starches, such as whole-grain products with all their nutrition, should be eaten in limited quantities and with other foods. Sugar should be completely avoided, as should stimulants; sugar, alcohol, coffee, and colas trigger the condition.

Labels on food containers must be read carefully. It is essential to avoid canned, packaged, or frozen foods with sugar, corn syrup, sucrose, dextrose, honey, or the like. This is vital. If not done, one can unwittingly undermine the whole effect of the rest of the diet. Important details on the diet are explained in a number of books. Several books that have been helpful to laymen in understanding and correcting hypoglycemia are listed in the recommended reading list at the end of this book.

Chapter 23

Alcoholism: A Vicious Cycle

"In the alcoholic—whether predisposed, active, or recovered—the prevailing factor is hypoglycemia." This is a summary provided by Dr. Harold W. Lovell and Dr. John W. Tintera for his lengthy article "The Prevailing Fact Is Hypoglycemia" in a 1966 issue of *Geriatrics*.

The most plausible answer I have been given from specialists in hypoglycemia is the following: when a person's blood sugar is frequently low, he learns, sometimes subconsciously, that if he eats something containing sugar or a stimulant he feels better. What he doesn't realize is that he has thereby set himself up for a rapid drop in his blood sugar levels later. When the drop comes, the natural thing to do, of course, is to eat some more of the sugar. Before long, he is living from one cola, piece of candy, or cup of coffee to another—year after year, with increasing damage to his system. This is the life style of many Americans. We have become physiologically dependent upon sugar and caffeine. We are addicted. We are sugarholics.

The reason the person who has eaten the sugar feels better (temporarily) is that his supply of blood sugar has (temporarily) been brought up to adequate levels. Any rapidly absorbed carbohydrate will do the same. Alcohol, for example. Therefore, instead of reaching for their coffee or sweet, some people reach for their beer, bourbon, or vodka. The drop which follows, however, can be precipitous and nerve-wracking. They begin to fear they can't cope. A legitimate fear, given the fact that their cells and brains are starving and their sugar processing mechanisms are being over-taxed. Another drink, however, steadies them again—for a while. Unfortunately, in quantity alcohol intoxicates while colas, coffee, and candy do not; so there are different and more serious consequences for the person who tries to keep himself going on alcohol.

Is Alcoholism Inherited?

Many alcoholics, recovered alcoholics, and people working with them believe that alcoholism tends to run in families. They see it in their parents and other close relatives. It is estimated that four out of five alcoholics have an alcoholic parent. Naturally, they are especially concerned that their children may succumb to this debilitating, and perhaps inevitable, disease. However, the actual connections which make alcoholism inheritable have always been obscure. Now they are more clear. In learning about hypoglycemia, we can see an understandable connection. It may be the hypoglycemia which is inheritable, an actual systemic tendency which, of course, can be inherited just as other systemic malfunctions can. What a great encouragement to the alcoholic or recovered alcoholic parent to know that there are definite measures that can be taken to decrease the possibility of his or her children going the alcoholic route!

Whether their hypoglycemia is inherited or induced, alcoholics often exhibit many of the standard symptoms associated with hypoglycemia, sometimes in rather severe form. Many crave sweets, for example, as well as stimulants and starches: colas, coffee, bread, spaghetti, potatoes, and rice; some alcoholics and recovered alcoholics can consume the most unbelievable amounts of any one of these at one sitting.

Given all we have considered above, we can understand how drinking gets out of control. It may not be a matter of will power. The fact is, some individuals simply cannot tolerate living with this endocrine imbalance and with the gruesome tricks it plays upon their reason and will. It is a horrible experience compounded by other people's misunderstanding, moral accusations, disgust, and abandonment.

Diet and Alcoholism

Dr. Cheraskin writes of experiments which indicate that diet can create alcoholism. One of the tests he cites was made at Loma Linda University in California. He relates that investigators induced a craving for alcohol in rats by feeding them a diet high in refined carbohydrates, low in vitamins, minerals, and proteins. He said:

> The rats were not psychologically stressed; they were not raised by "mean parents," but they turned eagerly to drink when deprived of proper diet.

> Thirty rats were divided into three groups for a sixteen week study. One group remained on the high-carbohydrate diet; another group ate the same diet supplemented with vitamins and minerals; and a third group consumed a balanced human diet.

> The result?

> Given a choice between plain drinking water and a 10 percent solution of ethyl alcohol, the rats on the high-carbohydrate diet drank, on an average, fifty milliliters— the equivalent of what would be a quart of 100-proof whiskey a day for an adult man. The rats on the fortified high-carbohydrate diet drank only one-third as much alcohol, while those on the well-balanced human diet generally preferred plain water.

> Dietary manipulation can turn teetotalers into alcoholics. Twenty percent of a group of rats maintained on a high-carbohydrate diet for five weeks did not develop a taste for alcohol until sugar was added to the solution. These rats then turned into the heaviest drinkers of all. When switched onto a balanced diet, they gradually became ex-alcoholics.[1]

Another test of great interest was made at the same university to determine whether a typical "teen-age diet," known to be nutritionally *marginal* rather than totally deficient, could also cause a craving for alcohol in rats. "Each rat was allowed a choice of drinking a solution composed of 10 percent alcohol and 90 percent water or simply plain water. Their basic diet consisted of glazed doughnuts, sweetened soft rolls, hot dogs, carbonated beverages, spaghetti and meatballs, apple pie and chocolate cake, white bread, green beans, tossed salad, candy and cookies.... the rats tippled freely. They drank even more when coffee or caffeine was added. Adding vitamin supplementation greatly reduced alcohol intake." [2]

Dr. Cheraskin concludes that "Experiments like these reinforce the idea of metabolic control mechanism, sensitive to dietary factors, that creates a *biologic thirst* for alcohol. They also offer some rationale for the ever-rising alcohol problem that educators have decried among high school and college students." [3] Much to our horror, we learn that drinking has become a serious problem among thirteen-year-olds today.

Proper Treatment

What, then, is the proper treatment? Alcoholism is a complex disease. It should not be oversimplified. Poor nutrition and hypoglycemia, however, do provide a physiological basis for many cases of alcoholism; for most cases, some doctors believe. There can be other causes as well; some of these may be psychological. Having hypoglycemia and being alcoholic can generate psychological and other problems, even if these problems did not exist before the disease developed.

Therefore, it is essential that each case be treated individually. For some, good nutrition, the hypoglycemia diet, plus no alcohol, will recoup vigorous health and confident, effective functioning. For others, the diet should be coupled with counseling and perhaps other kinds of therapy. Whatever the complications and contributing factors, however, we are told that there can be little progress, merely frustration, if the physiological factors are not dealt with directly and corrected.

Alcoholics Anonymous

Alcoholic Anonymous has done a unique and extremely effective job working with alcoholics. Nutritionists believe their contributions could be inestimably greater, however, if they would circulate a sensible diet for their members and inquirers. Their assistance would be still more significant if they would provide decaffeinated coffee (if the idea of coffee helps) and health-enhancing beverages at their meetings instead of their gallons of ordinary coffee, and if they would see the wisdom of furnishing cheese cubes or nuts or milk. When their members are at a meeting, many of them have not eaten for some time; therefore, their blood sugar levels are dropping. The protein snack would help break the cycle and contribute to a greater sense of well being, and it would certainly help avoid the drop in the blood sugar level the members experience when they have their usual coffee.

I am told that A.A. has a policy of introducing nothing outside its own program, and I appreciate their reasons for this. However, it does seem that anything as routine and necessary to life as eating could be mentioned in their literature, and that anything as detrimental to recovery as coffee and sugar could be eliminated.

I cannot stress too much that anyone who has alcoholism in his family and who finds himself frequently taking colas, coffee, sweets, beer, or other alcoholic beverages should realize that a trap may lie ahead for him—the trap of alcoholism. A.A. explains that alcohol is cunning, baffling, and powerful. Anyone who has these habits, therefore, should study nutrition and go on the hypoglycemia diet immediately. This would be a small price to pay for freedom from the agony of alcoholism. Furthermore, of course, the diet contributes significantly to excellent health in general.

Some doctors, and nutritionists of course, believe that supplemental vitamins and minerals are needed in recovering from alcohol addiction, and after recovery as well. Megavitamin doses of niacin, for example, are now being used in a number of rehabilitation centers and, I hope, will be used more widely and with more understanding. Deficiencies have developed in most Americans due to poor eating habits and devitalized foods, but especially in the alcoholic whose eating and drinking habits are often particularly inadequate and harmful. Dr. Roger J. Williams has written a small, easily read and instructive book entitled *Alcoholism, The Nutritional Approach.* This book suggests important guidelines for the alcoholic, the problem drinker, and the concerned parent, friend, and counselor.

There are other valuable pamphlets and books on alcohol-

ism available through Alcoholics Anonymous and Alcohol Information Centers, both of which are found in most cities and
are listed in telephone directories.

Alcoholics Anonymous offers additional help for the
spouse and children of alcoholics, for families of alcoholics are
in need of help too. They need help in knowing how to handle
the alcoholic; so often those nearest the alcoholic are unwittingly doing the very thing that makes the condition worse. They
also need to know how to preserve their own health and equi-
librium in the midst of their stress.

George Gallup reports that 12% of the families in our
country have a problem with alcohol. He also informs us that
alcoholism or excessive drinking is believed to be related to half
of the nation's traffic fatalities, half of the homicides, and a
third of the suicides.[4]

The alcoholics, the families and friends of alcoholics, and
the nation need all the help they can get to meet this problem.
Turning to A.A., which was founded by a Christian and is
based on turning one's will and life over to God, is the first step.
Good nutrition, including recognition of possible hypoglycemia, is the next.

PART 7

Nutrition As Christian Stewardship

So whether you eat or drink or whatever you do, do it all for the glory of God.

1 Corinthians 10:31

Chapter 24

The Predicament

In the previous chapters we have considered the discouraging predicament facing Americans today. We have the most abundant supply of food in the world and the most efficient means of distributing it to everyone. We have created powerful agencies to ensure that our food is honestly represented to us and free from harmful substances. Furthermore, we spend countless millions of dollars in food research. Yet for some reason, whenever we read a label, we sense that our food is not what it should be.

We also have thousands of highly trained doctors, extremely sophisticated medical facilities, and medical research programs supported by millions of dollars. Yet for some reason we really don't feel well. And we see much evidence that many other people aren't feeling well either.

We are dissatisfied with our food and we don't feel as well as we would like to because the people we pay to protect and promote our health—in other words, governmental agencies and food industries—are doing things which are actually detrimental to our health.

Our Neglect

We have allowed the food and beverage industries to convert us from God's natural provisions to their own highly processed and synthetic concoctions. Our tastes have been so perverted that we have forgotten how real food tastes. Our reasoning has become so distorted that we allow advertisements to persuade us that refined, depleted, processed foods and beverages, full of chemical additives, modified starch, imitation flavor, imitation color and sugar, are superior to real food.

We are a nation under God, governed by the people for the people, but we neglect to apprise ourselves of what government bureaucracies are allowing to happen to our food supply, and hence to our health. We blindly accept their approval of medicated feed for livestock and poultry. We seldom question their approval of fertilizers which are lacking important elements or their approval of pesticides which contain, and convey, poisons. We do not insist that they prohibit agri-business from using artificial techniques to deceive consumers into believing that their produce is fresh and ripe when it is not. Nor do we object when "more than one thousand chemicals which are regularly added to our food ... have never been tested for their potential to cause cancer, birth defects, or gene damage." [1] Technology is rapidly breaking down the basic structure of plant and animal life in many ways, and we haven't asked whether science is monitoring the results of these basic changes in health to the human being.

No Restrictions on Sugar

Our government for years has spent millions of dollars subsidizing sugar, and that sugar goes into many of our foods. A surprising amount of it goes into baby foods. Gerber, Heinz, and Beechnut refuse to disclose exactly how much sugar is added to their baby foods,[2] and they get away with it. Consumption of sugar-laden snacks has increased approximately 80% in the last three decades. Each American now consumes an average of eighteen pounds of candy each year.

Snacks and candy are often sold through vending machines. This source of pollution did a $5,000,000,000 business in 1973. Even dental schools have candy vendors in student lounges. A recent survey revealed that twenty-two of thirty-nine schools questioned had candy machines.[3] A petition was submitted to the government which would require vending contractors to stock at least half of each food vending machine with nutritious items. The petition was submitted by the Center for Science in the Public Interest, with the support of fifteen other groups and both Dr. Jean Mayer, nutritionist at Harvard, and Dr. George Briggs, nutritionist at the University of California. It was submitted to the General Services Administration which is supposed to promote programs that will improve the public's health. The response to the petition was minimal.[4]

The Center for Science in the Public Interest recently petitioned for the establishment of a standard of quality for breakfast cereals. The standard would set an acceptable level of sugar in cereals at 10% and would require a sugar content disclosure and warning labels on cereals containing more sugar. The FDA rejected the petition on the grounds that the agency had no information regarding the adverse effects of sugar consumption on health.[5] Goodness! Where have they been?

Inadequate Drug Restrictions

The Food and Drug Administration, therefore, together with the food industries, are not as concerned as they should be about food processing, artificial additives, and sugar. Nor is the Food and Drug Administration, together with the drug industries, as strict as it should be about the testing, marketing, and administration of drugs. We hear from doctors, pharmacologists, and other reliable sources that half of the antibiotics given in hospitals are either not needed or incorrectly prescribed,[6] and that prescription drugs are responsible for over 100,000 unnecessary deaths a year.[7] In other words, adverse drug reactions kill more victims than does breast cancer in women. It is estimated further that 30 to 40% of all hospital patients suffer adverse reactions.[8] Many drugs which have been allowed on the market have been forced off because of adverse, even fatal, side-effects. Furthermore, countless over-the-counter drugs are permitted in unlimited quantities; for example, fifty tons of aspirin are consumed by Americans daily.

We can see from the above, and I think each of us knows

from our own experience, that we have been indoctrinated regarding the benefits of crisis medicine and the drugs upon which it is based. As a result, we have overlooked the soundness and the necessity of preventive medicine. We are unaware that the correction of biochemical deficiency and imbalance with the natural elements God designed for our bodies is the prerequisite for healing and abundant health.

Need for More Awareness of Orthomolecular Psychiatry

Our predicament, as pointed out in earlier chapters, has another important dimension. We are told that one out of three families has a problem of serious mental illness and that number is increasing. We also hear that mental retardation is increasing. Furthermore, we know that doctors and psychiatrists still rely upon drugs, shock therapy, and psychotherapy with disappointing results, even aggravated conditions in some cases. Along with all of this, we know that individuals in the medical profession have their own problems with alcohol, drugs, neurosis, and suicide. There is some evidence that physicians are more likely than most people to become addicted to narcotics. Yet, most doctors and psychiatrists have overlooked orthomolecular psychiatry, a thoroughly researched approach based on vitamin-mineral therapy which has resulted in outstanding work in mental, emotional, alcohol, and drug problems.

Critical Role of Preventive Medicine

Our predicament is the result of the convergence of many forces. Government agencies, food and drug industries, and health professions, because they still dismiss preventive medicine and orthomolecular psychiatry, do not appreciate the critical role of nutrition. Because government agencies and the food industry still lack genuine commitment to the consumer, the daily diet of most Americans has become a major cause of ill-health and degenerative disease. We learn from responsible sources that our nation's diet is the direct cause, or a significant contributing cause, of numerous debilitating conditions. Among them are anemia, weight problems, severe dental and oral problems, behavior and mental and emotional problems, diabetes, hypoglycemia, coronary ills, alcoholism, appendicitis, diverticulitis, irritation of the upper alimentary canal, esophagus, stomach, and duodenum, and even cancer.

Is there any hope?

Chapter 25

The Promise

I think we can be encouraged about a change for the better in our nation's diet. Actually, only a small percentage of people may be eating truly nutritious food, but it is a beginning and the number is growing.

Other signs of progress are the excellent and well-documented books and articles on various aspects of food which are appearing in increasing numbers. Natural food cookbooks are also on the increase, and natural food stores and restaurants are developing; some colleges and universities are now providing health food meals in their dining rooms. There is growing interest in methods of organic gardening and farming, and there is the wonderful fact that the natural foods orientation is strongest among young people—our future leaders, doctors, ministers, businesspeople, and politicians. We can look to our young people for the generation by generation awareness and change that must come if we are to survive.

Encouraging Examples of Progress

An example of what is happening in a small way, and in different ways around the country, is a group which met in Freeport, Illinois, to educate others on what is happening to the quality of our food. The Freeport paper gives an account of the Junior Women's Guild at the YWCA which gave a program with the clever title "Guess What's Coming to Dinner." Their plea was to read labels. The speaker recited a typical child's menu for one day and wrote out all the ingredients. More than 230 of the ingredients were additives![1]

We can be encouraged that the facts about the damage sugar does to our health are bursting the bonds of suppression and are now being heard. In a comprehensive review in *The New York Review of Books* entitled "Death for Dinner," Daniel Zwerdling covered several pertinent books dealing with food as well as some of the hearings before the Senate Select Committee on Nutrition and Human Needs.[2] Zwerdling points out that the evidence implicating sugar presented at an international convention of scientists in West Germany was so strong that people were urged to stop eating it. Such a recommendation from international scientists may not influence our government, but it can have a significant impact on the people of our country.

Some people are being influenced. We see it now in small isolated changes, and it is these changes which, when multiplied across the country, can eventually turn the tide for better nutrition. For example, the food editor of a paper in Phoenix ran an article discouraging the use of sugar and giving recipes with healthful sweeteners. And we are hearing more and more about local "bake-offs" where healthful ingredients have been used; for example, honey is used instead of sugar.

The soaring sugar prices have occasioned the publication of healthful, as well as economically helpful, ways to substitute for sugar, For instance, one syndicated newspaper service circulated an article entitled "Sugar Price Hike Called a Boon to Health." It quoted Dr. Abraham Nizel, professor of Nutrition and Preventive Medicine at Tufts University, who said that "if sugar were eliminated from the diet it would be one of the greatest boons in the nation's history." [3] Dr. Michael Jacobson, of Washington's Center for the Science in the Public Interest, agrees: "It's unfortunate it took high prices to convince Americans they shouldn't eat sugar but if that's what it takes, I'm all for it."

The sugar price hike also brought suggestions for ways to

cut costs in baking by reducing the use of sugar. This should show our bakers that sugar is not as necessary to their business as they had assumed. "There are approximately 50,000,000 one-pound loaves of bread produced each day in our country; these contain 3,000,000 pounds of sugar. For this sugar, the sugar in their bread alone, Americans pay $2,000,000 a day." [4]

Some people are doing a great deal to educate the public regarding the dangers of sugar and the value of products made without it. An example is the Consumer Awareness Program of the Office of Economic Opportunity in New Mexico. The program is sponsoring a "Sugar-less Snack" cookbook contest, and special emphasis is being given to local ethnic foods. The program also publishes a "Sugar-less Snack Newsletter." [5]

We are now hearing the truth about sugar consumption from both international and local sources. We need no longer live under the illusion that sugar is a necessary source of energy to the body in the concentrated form in which it is manufactured. It is not good for us; it is not a harmless product with which to enhance the flavor of our foods.

Further Findings in Caffeine

Other foods, besides sugar, are receiving critical attention —coffee, for example. Dr. Marshall Mandell, director of the New England Foundation of Allergic and Environmental Disease, dealt with coffee in a seminar at the International Academy of Preventive Medicine. Thousands of adults have been tested, and he believes that coffee is the reason for many of their physical and mental ills. In fact, he considers coffee to be the number one offender. Caffeine is only one of the problems of this complex brew, and we are told that decaffeinated coffee only brings more chemicals into our diet: the chemicals used to remove the caffeine.

Dr. John Greden, of Walter Reed Medical Center, spoke about the effect of caffeine at a recent meeting of the American Psychiatric Association. He reported that his research indicates a link between caffeine and anxiety. Too much caffeine, he explained, can cause symptoms which include nervousness, irritability, lethargy, insomnia, and headaches. It can also cause heart palpitations, irregular heartbeats, and skin flushing. In the intestinal tract, too much caffeine can produce nausea, diarrhea, vomiting, and pain. However, coffee and colas are not the only things which contain caffeine in substantial amounts. Dr. Greden informs us that it is found in cocoa and many pain killers as well.

Physicians consider that 250 milligrams of caffeine constitute a large amount. Ten to twelve cups of coffee a day total 1000 milligrams. On this basis, more than two cups a day, or less than two cups with colas or pain relievers during the day, constitute a large amount of caffeine. Mandell and many nutritionists consider that any amount of coffee or cola is too much and should be avoided entirely. We may not like to hear these findings, but we can be encouraged because we can now make our choice on the basis of fact, not on fiction or acquired taste.

Recent studies of Mormons and Seventh Day Adventists are of interest. Dr. James E. Enstrom of the School of Public Health at the University of California has found that among the Mormons, who shun alcohol, tobacco, and coffee, there are half as many cases of cancer than among others in California. Utah (the Mormon state where many Mormons have even further dietary restrictions) has the lowest incidence of cancer of any state in the union. Dr. Roland L. Phillips of Loma Linda University has found this is also true of the Seventh Day Adventists who observe dietary restrictions.[6]

Vitamin-Mineral Therapy

Also promising, extremely promising, is the continuing research on vitamin-mineral therapy and the reports coming in from many parts of the world. For instance, the reports from a prominent Swedish doctor on controlled studies using vitamin E in vascular surgery indicate that with extra vitamin E in the muscles, walking can become a pleasure again for those with obstructed leg arteries; blood flow increases and the chances of losing a limb diminish greatly.[7] We recall that the Drs. Shute of Canada have been seeing these kinds of results in their patients for many years. Now it seems that every few months we hear more from other reliable doctors and researchers concerning the beneficial results being obtained from the use of vitamin E. But the point is, there are groups which are always forging ahead in research here and in other parts of the world regardless of the negative attitudes of others. Progress on vitamin-mineral therapy of all kinds is definitely being realized.

Increased Awareness of Natural Foods

The health food orientation is, indeed, taking hold. The cereal and bread industries, for instance, are feeling the trend enough to attempt to turn out their own "health" products in competition with those in the health food stores. Their motive for health is questionable; most of their products are anything but healthful. Also most of the "natural" cereals produced by the large manufacturers are not all that natural. Some contain white sugar and brown sugar. Unfortunately the manufacturers think, or they think the public thinks, that brown sugar is more natural and healthier than white sugar. Of course, it is not. It is just as harmful and unnecessary. Some cereals boast "no additives" when they do have an additive: sugar. However, regardless of the motive, we see evidence of progress when large corporations want to capitalize on the trend by selling to the "health food nuts." This is a definite indication that significant number of Americans are waking up to their need for better nutrition. Nutritionists are finally being heard to some degree.

The Truth Is Coming Through

Doctors who are making important discoveries regarding the relationship between what we eat, our ills, and our behavior are also finally being heard. For example, Dr. Ben Feingold's important work on the relationship between food additives and hyperkinesis was criticized and discounted for two years by the FDA. Feingold says that the FDA had been like a "brick wall, giving me no support, only discouragement, as though they were representatives of the food industry rather than a government agency." [8] Nevertheless, his work was appreciated by many doctors and certainly by thousands of citizens. Enough people in the country have now heard about Dr. Feingold's work so that Washington has been forced to take note.

Unfortunately, we all know that Feingold's experience with the FDA, when it acted like a representative of the food industry, is not singular. We have learned, too, that we can no longer trust the FDA's sanction of the safety of additives being used. As Zwerdling recounts in his review "Death for Dinner,"

"Most eaters once assumed that synthetic additives in food must be safe but recent evidence has caused that kind of blind trust to crack." [9] People are beginning to hear about what is happening to our food supply, and that does make a difference in Washington.

Such organizations as the Federation of Homemakers and the Center of Science in the Public Interest have sought out facts, brought much information to light, and brought pressure to bear in Washington. Furthermore, the attempt by the FDA to limit the potencies of vitamin supplements brought letters from thousands of citizens. These are some of the reasons why Congress has been spurred into action. The Senate Select Committee on Nutrition and Human Needs has heard evidence from distinguished and independent scientists on what is happening to our food supply and on the individual's right to purchase supplementation in whatever potency he finds important to his well being.

Congressmen Are Taking a Stand

Individual members of Congress are also beginning to investigate the condition of our food. This is most encouraging. Senator Richard Schweiker of Pennsylvania contends that we take better care of our cars than our bodies and that our national health is at stake. He sponsored the "Nutritional Medical Act of 1973" to encourage nutritional education courses in medical schools and the "Nutritional Labeling Act of 1973" to require the labeling of all food commodities with their nutritional value. Recently Senator McGovern of South Dakota has proposed an independent office of nutrition in the federal government. It is encouraging that occasionally, at least, there is interaction between qualified scientists and nutritionists from outside the government and members of Congress. It is a step in the right direction—an important step.

We remember Senator Proxmire's statement that the FDA "in their zeal and hostility had thrown up a group of strawmen, distorted statements and outright misstatements of facts and scientific evidence." We should also remember his statement that "the FDA had been turning out propaganda for years in their attempt to smear the health food industry." We can take heart because this sort of information is coming to light. It affects how we vote and what letters we write to Congress. It also puts us on notice about the campaign against health foods.

Competency Within the FDA

We must not forget however, that the FDA does have competent doctors and research chemists who do not go along with many of the decisions the FDA makes or with its failures to protect the consumer adequately. Jean Verrett, a former research chemist with the FDA, corroborates this in her book *Eating May Be Hazardous to Your Health.*

Strength was shown on a FDA review panel, chaired by Dr. Nicholas Hightower, when it did not defer to the drug industry. Because of its findings the country is being alerted to the harm caused by over-the-counter laxatives which are used for longer than a week. Hightower maintains that anti-diarrhetics are either harmful or ineffective. When asked on nationwide television what Americans should use in place of laxatives and anti-diarrhetics, he explained that these bowel problems are generally the result of eating synthetic foods which are low in residue; his recommendation, therefore, is to maintain a diet having fiber.

Definite Progress

There are great future possibilities in the fields of nutrition and preventive medicine. Dr. Roger Williams envisions one: a computerized record of each newborn baby's biochemical pattern will be one of the obstetrical services of hospitals. This analysis will serve as a basis for future nurture and treatment. Williams thinks it is highly probable that many of the individual "leanings," which make us all susceptible to some diseases and resistant to others, can be determined at that time and some cases with special nutritional needs can be treated, thereby obviating future trouble. Williams says, "We will deemphasize the use of medicine and we will concentrate on constructive measures—providing the cells and tissues of our bodies with the best possible nutritional environment." [10]

We can certainly be encouraged about the growing interest in nutrition and preventive medicine. Nutritional societies made up of doctors, nutritionists, biochemists as well as men and women of other disciplines, are growing. The effort must expand. Dr. Jean Mayer said on nationwide television that there must be a massive effort in nutritional education for preventive medicine.[11] Senator Schweiker exhorts us: "We should not just treat medical problems after they have already become serious, but should use nutritional dietary practices as a key means of preventing these medical problems from arising in the first place." [12] In other words, the relationship which exists between what we eat now and how we will feel in the future is coming through. We can be encouraged that it is coming from more and more quarters: professional, scientific, political, and domestic.

We can take heart, then, in the midst of our nutritional predicament. The evidence of progress is indeed exhilarating. More books and articles are being prepared and published, and more natural food stores and restaurants are being established. Interest is growing rapidly in organic gardening and farming. Young people are taking exciting initiatives. Productive research is continuing despite opposition. Medical practice is opening to new dimensions. The dangers of certain foods are being exposed. We are being represented in Washington by well-informed groups of volunteers, and some members of Congress are investigating and taking stands for sound nutrition.

There are more exciting developments taking place. Granted, most information is not being widely publicized and most people are not paying attention, but a start has been made. The movement is underway and growing. The future holds promise for better health and stronger bodies with which to serve the Lord in whatever ways we are called.

Chapter 26

The Practice

It is time we stop defending the good job we think we are doing for our family, church, or Christian group and find out whether we really are so knowledgeable. We must stop thinking we know all we need to know about food and start reading up on the subject. We have to stop thinking we are a healthy nation and face the reality that we are not. We must stop believing the advertisements and start considering how we really feel and look. We have got to realize how serious a responsibility it is to feed people, especially when most of society is conditioned to eating poorly.

It is a serious responsibility to feed people: our family, our friends, ourselves. And it is, for the Christian, an incomparable opportunity. Feeding the body is a ministry. We have examples of Jesus ministering with food—good food. When He fed the multitudes, He fed them on high-quality protein in fish and the staff of life, whole-grain bread (Matt. 14:19). Howard Butt, in his compelling and poignantly relevant book for the Christian, says that "Christianity is not a way of doing special things. It is a special way of doing everything."[1] I believe this, and I believe that it includes a special way of caring for our bodies.

Abolish Nutritional Illiteracy

If we are serious about caring for our bodies in special ways, the first step is to start reading, "There is a need to abolish nutritional illiteracy," Dr. Roger Williams urges. "Nutritional information needs to filter down." [2] A number of books have been suggested in previous chapters and at the end of the book. It would be helpful to start with these. There are many other books and articles, and more appearing every month.

The second step is to find a good nutritionist. I know of nothing more important to our physical well-being than to have a competent nutritionist. If we do not, we must read books on nutrition which are written for the layman by competent men and women in the field. Also, we would be wise not to be side-tracked by the books of cultists, faddists, and self-appointed food specialists. We want to accumulate a general knowledge of good nutrition for ourselves and our families until we find a professional to advise us further.

The problem is, how do we find a competent nutritionist? The answer is to look for one who has had extensive formal training in biochemistry as well as clinical experience with knowledgeable doctors. It is the nutritionist with this background who is invaluable.

As discussed previously, each of us has our own biochemical individuality. We have inherited different biochemical constitutions and have been exposed to different environmental factors, both externally and internally. These, in turn, affect the cells of our bodies; we must furnish these cells with the particular elements they need, as well as reduce those elements which are in excess. Biochemical balance can only be determined and established by one who is both knowledgeable and experienced.

Clinical nutrition, then, is a great deal more than the diets of cultists, the formulas of faddists, or one person's idea of the best way to eat. It is also well beyond the knowledge of dieticians and home economists. It is even beyond the knowledge which we all should have about good, wholesome food and balanced meals. Clinical nutrition includes this, of course, but it also provides the expertise which can prevent or treat disease.

There are some doctors who have extensive knowledge of

cellular nutrition, but they are unique. The large majority have no training at all in it. It will be a great day when medical students study nutrition in medical school so their general advice is informed and their influence revolutionizes food management in hospitals. Beyond this, however, real expertise in nutrition is needed in daily medical practice. We all need nutritional check-ups. It could hardly be expected of many physicians to learn an entirely new field when there is more information than most can keep abreast of in his own field. Because cellular nutrition is a completely different approach to health than the medicinal and pharmaceutical approach, it is a difficult and time-consuming route, I am told, for a medical doctor to undertake. The solution obviously is a combination of disciplines if we are to have complete care and realize more abundant health. This kind of teamwork is found in isolated parts of the country, but where it is not, we are left on our own to find a competent nutritionist.

Our Responsibility to Others

So much for ourselves. What about our special care for the bodies of others? What about our churches and other Christian groups? Actually, I think we are ready to admit that we have done our share to detract from the responsibility of taking proper care of ourselves by not providing and eating really nourishing foods. We may therefore have put a "stumbling block or obstacle" in the way of a brother (Rom. 14:13).

If we believe that the care of the body is an act of Christian stewardship, then we Christians should lead the field in the practice of good nutrition. This means not only feeding ourselves and our families nutritiously, but also serving really nourishing foods at all our gatherings. It may sound disastrous —unthinkable—to change such traditions as potluck suppers, receptions, coffee hours, and bake sales, but it need not be. It could be our supreme opportunity. By beginning with the congregation, we could help improve the health of the nation. We, as Christians, have unique opportunities to educate one another and to witness to God's total, beautiful, healthful, and delicious provisions for mankind.

Is it too much to expect Christian schools, colleges, and seminaries to teach the normal process of health to their students and feed them the kind of food which will build strong bodies and contribute to their discipleship? Some institutions could no doubt grow their own food, and students and faculty might well learn a lot about themselves and creation in the process.

When Jesus said, "Feed the hungry," He certainly did not mean with food that would not adequately nourish the cells of the body. Lamentably, institutions go right along with the pollution of our food, thereby appearing to sanction it. Our institutions may not be able to bring about immediate change in our nation's air and water pollution, but they could do a great deal *immediately* toward eliminating our food pollution.

In addition to feeding young people wisely, Christian schools and other institutions might well encourage them to go on for formal training in biochemistry and nutrition. The need for competent people in this area is great. Research and knowledge are developing at ever-increasing rates, and it will undoubtedly be one of the exciting careers of the future.

I have been connected with the food business in a number of ways. My most recent experience came while I was co-director of a multiple restaurant which had fourteen kitchens representing nine nations. We fed up to 16,000 people a week. I know only too well what the average American eats, and I am well aware of how teen-agers feed themselves. But I also know that institutions, restaurants, and food stores can make available, and even feature, truly healthful foods. I also know that those of us who teach cooking, lecture on cooking, and write cookbooks can start including natural food recipes. Information can start "filtering down," as Dr. Roger Williams exhorts, in these ways, too. Williams says: "The kind of nutrition we crucially need, what the food industry should provide us, is *complete nutrition*—the kind that leads to abundant health." [3]

Our Depth of Conviction

If we do set out in a new direction, we will probably meet with opposition taking many forms and coming from many quarters. But there is always resistance to change, especially when it means changing one's habits. This is why each Christian must examine the predicament and the promise and then make his or her own evaluation and decision. It is only with personal conviction and God's help that any of us will be able to take hold and forge ahead—to change our personal lives and begin to change, where possible, our churches, businesses, professions, and government. Change within each of these areas, and within each of us, is essential. This change, however, will require a new depth of understanding. Dr. Ross Hume Hall expresses well the critical need for new understanding:

> Everyone to a greater or lesser degree adapts his personal lifestyle to the demands of a technical world. There are those who wish to modify that world in some way, to bring the technical system into rapport with the realities of nature and the spirit of man. Such deliberate change will not be easily accomplished without understanding the major forces flowing through society. Not to change is to risk the continued impoverishment of natural processes.[4]

Chapter 27

The Perspective

Finally, brothers, whatever is true, whatever is noble, whatever is right, whatever is pure, whatever is lovely, whatever is admirable—if anything is excellent or praiseworthy—think about such things.

Philippians 4:8

Is it possible that this portion of Scripture pertains to every area of our lives except how we nourish the temple of the Holy Spirit? I think not. I believe we are to "think about such things" by learning to select and prepare the food we allow to become our bodies.

If we let this and other portions of Scripture penetrate and illuminate every aspect of our lives (especially our most cherished daily habits), we may need some new searching of ourselves. What have we been eating since birth? How much have we been taking for granted? Where have we been correctly informed and where wrongly informed even by well-meaning people? What have we been feeding others at home, in church, in school, in business? Finally, and most importantly, how do the Scriptures and our commitment concern our bodies and the ways we sustain them?

Actually, the way in which the Christian perspective affects our eating habits does not have to do with us; it has to do with whom we contain. Jesus Christ said that He would dwell in us. We are His vessels. The integrity of the vessel is essential to that which it contains. Besides containing, we are to convey. Our faith, priorities, attitudes, as well as our bodies, do convey a message. In other words, we are the message. We are ambassadors for Christ. Are we the message He wants us to be?

Christ's message was that of love. It is a Christian's pleasure, therefore, to act in loving ways—to receive and give. Are we treating God's vessel, our body, with love when we receive that which does damage? And are we treating God's vessels with love when we give others that which is destructive? When we receive food from someone, we are allowing the person to contribute directly to our very substance, and when we prepare and give food to a person, we offer the gift which concretely becomes a part of that person. Feeding a person something which is beneficial helps sustain that person's life, but choosing and preparing food ignorantly engages us in a subtle form of violence.

We are privileged stewards of the earth's resources—our air and water, for example. This we are beginning to realize. What we have yet to realize is that we are privileged stewards of our own individual resources: our muscles, nerves, organs, cells, and biochemical processes. Once we grow into this awareness, we will appreciate more fully the reciprocal relationship between our planet's resources and our personal resources. For, in truth, our abuse of one (our air, for example) has detrimental effects upon the other (our lungs, for example). Similarly, our respect for and development of one contributes to an appreciation for and development of the other. Separation of our earth's resources and our individual resources results in a deterioration of both. Those things for which we are stewards cannot, therefore, be separated. God's entire creation has integrity.

As stewards we have been entrusted with the development and use of all our resources, technology, organizations, talents, and money. More particularly, we are entrusted with the development and use of our bodies. Because of our abundance and the access to knowledge we possess in our country, we have extraordinary opportunities to be good stewards. But we also have extraordinary power: power to construct or destroy.

Given the presence of Christ, given our awareness of our bodies and our new ability to nourish them, we have capacities to change more constructively and to contribute more fully than we realize. Our potential is unlimited. With our new appreciation for our bodies and our new understanding of proper nourishment, we can select, purchase, prepare, and serve food with new confidence and enthusiasm.

Beyond that, we as Christians can represent our new awareness, use our new knowledge, and enjoy our improved health according to the distinctive gifts we have been given. For some of us, teaching or writing may come most naturally. Others may find fulfillment by representing or persuading. A few relish the challenge of organizing, planning, and executing. Some are most creative when they are listening. Others are most communicative when they are providing a quiet example.

If we do "think about such things," perhaps we will develop sufficient wisdom to grasp this perspective and to commit ourselves with courage to complete wholeness.

So whether you eat or drink or whatever you do, do it all
for the glory of God.

1 Corinthians 10:31

Footnotes

Introduction

1. Paul Tournier, *Fatigue in Modern Society* (Richmond, Virginia: John Knox Press, 1965), p. 8.

Chapter 1

1. Alvin Toffler, *Future Shock* (New York: Bantam Books, 1970), pp. 36, 37.
2. Ross Hume Hall, *Food for Nought: The Decline of Nutrition* (New York: Medical Department, Harper and Row, new ed., 1974), p. VII.

Chapter 2

1. Weston A. Price, *Nutrition and Physical Degeneration* (Santa Monica, CA: Pottenger Foundation, Inc.), pp. XVII, XVIII.
2. Sir Robert Carrison, *Studies in Deficiency Diseases* (Reading, England: 5 Derby Road-Caversham).
3. Wilmon Menard, *Prevention*, January 1974.
4. Richard Passwater, *Supernutrition: The Megavitamin Revolution* (New York: The Dial Press, 1975), pp. 133, 134.
5. Wilfrid E. Shute and Harald Taub, *Vitamin E for Ailing and Healthy Hearts* (New York: Pyramid Publications, Inc., 1972), p. 7.

Chapter 3

1. Miles H. Robinson, *Executive Health,* vol. XI, no. 6.
2. T. L. Cleave, *The Saccharine Disease* (New Canaan, CT: Keats Publishing Co., 1975), p. 29.
3. David Reuben, *The Save Your Life Diet* (New York: Random House, 1975), p. 4.
4. Robinson, *Executive Health.*
5. T. R. Van Dellen, Syndicated Column, June 1973; Jean Mayer, Syndicated Column, August 1973.
6. Ray Wolfe, *Prevention,* June 1974.
7. Hall, *Food for Nought,* p. 24.
8. Catharyn Elwood, *Feel Like a Million* (New York: Pocket Books), p. 39.
9. William Dufty, *Sugar Blues* (Radnor, PA: Chilton Book Co., 1975), p. 109.
10. F. Earle Barcus, *Wall Street Journal,* 8 January 1976.
11. Jim Hightower, *Eat Your Heart Out: How Food Profiteers Victimize the Consumer* (New York: Crown Publishers, Inc., 1975), p. 40.

12. Jean Mayer, Syndicated Column, January 1976.
13. "More Facts on Good Nutrition: An Easy-to-Swallow Guide to Good Nutrition" (undated booklet), Sugar Information, General P.O. Box 94, New York, NY 10001.
14. James Trager, *Foodbook* (New York: Avon Books, 1970), p. 430.
15. John Yudkin, *Sweet and Dangerous* (New York: Bantam Books, Inc., 1972), chap. 9.
16. Ibid., p. 113.
17. Ibid., p. 141.
18. Ibid., p. 125.
19. Ibid., p. 130.
20. Ibid., chap. 13.
21. Ibid., p. 130.
22. Ibid., p. 58.
23. Ibid., p. 94.
24. Ibid., p. 95.
25. Ibid., p. 95.
26. Ibid., pp. 95, 96.
27. Ibid., p. 5.

Chapter 4

1. Jacqueline Verrett and Jean Carper, *Eating May Be Hazardous to Your Health* (New York: Simon and Schuster, Inc., 1974).
2. Michael F. Jacobson, *Eaters Digest: The Consumer Factbook of Food Additives* (New York: Doubleday and Co., 1972), p. 9.
3. James S. Turner, *The Chemical Feast: Report on the Food and Drug Administration* —Ralph Nader Study Group Reports (New York: Grossman Publisher, Inc., 1970), p. V.
4. Roger J. Williams, *Nutrition Against Disease* (New York: Pitman Publisher Corp., 1971), p. 207.
5. Beatrice Trum Hunter, *Consumer Beware!: Your Food and What's Been Done to It* (New York: Simon and Shuster, 1972), p. 82.
6. Beatrice Trum Hunter, *The Mirage of Safety* (Totowa, NJ: Charles Scribner's Sons, 1975).
7. Hunter, *Beware*, p. 82.
8. Harold Rosenberg and A. N. Feldzaman, *The Doctor's Book of Vitamin Therapy* (New York: G. P. Putnam's Sons, 1974), p. 69.
9. Hunter, *Beware*, pp. 93, 96, 97.
10. Hightower, *Eat Heart Out*, p. 88.
11. Verrett and Carper, *Eating Hazardous,* pp. 147, 148.
12. Ibid., p. 142.
13. Ibid., p. 146.
14. Hunter, *Beware*, pp. 60, 61.
15. Verrett and Carper, *Eating Hazardous,* p. 66.
16. Hightower, *Eat Heart Out*, p. 90.
17. Beatrice Trum Hunter, *The Natural Foods Primer* (New York: Simon and Schuster, 1972), p. 17.
18. Verrett and Carper, *Eating Hazardous,* p. 213.
19. Nikki and David Goldbeck, *The Supermarket Handbook: Access to Whole Foods* (New York: Harper and Row Publishers, Inc., 1973), p. 245.

Chapter 5

1. Gene Marine and Judith Van Allen, *Food Pollution: The Violation of Our Inner Ecology* (New York: Holt, Rinehart and Winston, 1972), p. 248.
2. Ibid., p. 249.
3. Hightower, *Eat Heart Out*, p. 40.
4. Bernard and Joeva Bellew, "An M.D.'s Defense of Raw Milk," *Let's Live*, July 1974.
5. Ibid.
6. Ibid.
7. Ibid.
8. Goldbeck, *Supermarket*, p. 26.

Chapter 6

1. Hall, *Food Nought*, p. 141.
2. Elwood, *Feel Like Million*, p. 264.
3. Robert Rodale, *Prevention*, April 1974.
4. Frank A. Gilbert, *Mineral Nutrition and the Balance of Life* (Norman, Oklahoma: University of Oklahoma Press, 1957), quoted by Robert Rodale, *Prevention*, April 1974.
5. Colin Fisher, *Let's Live*, July 1974.
6. *Organic Gardening*, August 1974.
7. Jean Dye Gassow, *Nutrition Today*, March/April 1974.
8. Hunter, *Beware*, p. 112.
9. Hall, *Food Nought*, p. 83.
10. Ibid., p. 85.
11. Ibid., p. 86.
12. Verrett and Carper, *Eating Hazardous*, pp. 167, 168.
13. Ibid., p. 175.
14. *U.S. News and World Report*, 23 February 1976.
15. Verrett and Carper, *Eating Hazardous*, p. 176.
16. Ibid., p. 177.
17. Hunter, *Beware*, p. 158.
18. Goldbeck, *Supermarket*, p. 56.
19. Beatrice Trum Hunter, ed., *Food and Your Health* —Consumers' Research (New Canaan, CT: Keats Publishing, Inc., 1974), pp. 72, 74.
20. John McClure, *Meat Eaters Are Threatened* (New York: Pyramid Publications, Inc., 1973).
21. Hightower, *Eat Heart Out*, p. 98.
22. Ibid., pp. 98, 99.
23. Ibid., p. 99.
24. Ibid., p. 99.
25. *Nutrition News* quoted by Ross Hume Hall, *Food Nought*, p. 55.
26. *New Science* quoted by Ross Hume Hall, *Food Nought*, pp. 55, 56.
27. Hall, *Food Nought*, p. 56.
28. Jean Mayer, Syndicated Column, 12 March 1973.
29. Goldbeck, *Supermarket*, p. 54.

Chapter 7

1. Williams, *Against Disease,* p. 13.

Chapter 8

1. Emanuel Cheraskin is Chairman of the Department of Oral Medicine at the University of Alabama School of Dentistry. He holds degrees in both medicine and dentistry, is consultant to several professional groups in the field of nutrition, and has written several books.

Chapter 9

1. Williams, *Against Disease,* p. 51.

Chapter 10

1. Passwater, *Supernutrition,* p. 46.
2. Ibid., p. 46.
3. Ibid., p. 50.

Chapter 13

1. Passwater, *Supernutrition,* pp. 86, 87.
2. Joan Libman, *Wall Street Journal,* 15 May 1975.
3. Robert Fletcher Alhen, *Let's Live,* April 1974.
4. Emanuel Cheraskin, William Ringsdorf, et. al., *Psycho-Dietetics: Food as the Key to Emotional Health* (New York: Stein and Day Publishers, 1974), p. 165.
5. Ibid., pp. 164, 165.
6. Passwater, *Supernutrition,* p. 75.
7. Ibid., p. 76.
8. Cheraskin and Ringsdorf, *Psycho-Dietetics,* p. 165.
9. Passwater, *Supernutrition,* p. 80.
10. Denton Cooley, *House and Garden Magazine,* June 1974.
11. Passwater, *Supernutrition,* p. 82.
12. Cheraskin and Ringsdorf, *Psycho-Dietetics,* p. 165.
13. Ibid., p. 165.

Chapter 14

1. William Robbins, *The American Food Scandal* (Caldwell, NJ: William Morrow and Company, Inc., 1974), p. 3.
2. Jacobson, *Eaters Digest,* p. 14.

3. United Press International, December 1974.
4. Charles H. Spurgeon, *Morning and Evening* (Grand Rapids, MI: Zonder-van Publishing House, 1955).

Chapter 15

1. Dufty, *Blues,* p. 122.
2. Ibid., pp. 129, 130.

Chapter 16

1. *Washington Post,* 5 November 1971.

Chapter 17

1. Roger Williams, *Nutrition in a Nutshell* (New York: Doubleday and Co., 1972), pp. 50, 51.
2. Price, *Physical Degeneration.*
3. Cheraskin and Ringsdorf, *Psycho-Dietetics,* p. 31.
4. Toffler, *Shock,* p. 20.
5. Williams, *Nutrition in Nutshell,* p. 7.
6. Price, *Physical Degeneration.*
7. Margaret E. Kenda and Phyliss S. Williams, *The Natural Baby Food Cookbook* (New York: Avon Books, 1973), p. 3.
8. Ibid., pp. 1, 2.
9. Ibid., p. 3.
10. Ibid., p. 4.
11. Ibid., pp. 6, 12.
12. Roger Williams, Seminar of International Academy of Preventive Medicine, October 1973.
13. Jeanne Lesem, United Press International, 21 August 1974.

Chapter 18

1. Jean Mayer, Syndicated Column, 12 March 1973.

Chapter 20

1. Dorothea Van Gundy Jones, *The Soybean Cookbook* (New York: Gramercy Publishing House, 1963), p. 11.
2. Cheraskin and Ringsdorf, *Psycho-Dietetics,* pp. 165, 166.
3. *Seeds and Sprouts for Life* (Solano Beach, CA: Bernard Jensen Products Publishing Division), p. 1.

230

Chapter 21

1. Shute and Taub, *Ailing and Healthy Hearts,* p. 40.
2. Ibid., p. 179.
3. Ibid., pp. 44, 45.
4. Ibid., p. 46.
5. Rosenberg and Feldzaman, *Doctor's Vitamin Therapy,* p. 132.
6. Ibid., pp. 135, 136.
7. Ibid., p. 137.
8. Linda Clark, *Know Your Nutrition* (New Canaan, CT: Keats Publishing Co., 1973), p. 130.
9. Ibid., p. 129.
10. Cheraskin and Ringsdorf, *Psycho-Dietetics,* pp. 121, 122.
11. Harold Rosenberg, *Healthline,* December 1975.
12. William Proxmire, *Let's Live,* August 1974, pp. 63–65.
13. Congressional Record, (93rd Congress—First Session), vol. 119, no. 195, 12 December 1973.
14. Milton Silverman and Philip R. Lee, *Pills, Profits, and Politics* (Berkeley, CA: University of California Press, 1974) quoted by Nicholas Von Hoffman, "Legal Overkill: The Deadly Dangers of Prescription Drugs," *Arizona Republic,* 7 June 1974.

Chapter 22

1. H. J. Roberts, *The Causes, Ecology and Prevention of Traffic Accidents: With Emphasis Upon Traffic Medicine, Epidemiology, Sociology, and Logistics* (Springfield, IL: Charles C. Thomas, 1971), quoted by Mark Bricklin, "Sugar Unmasked as Highway Killer," *Prevention,* March 1972.
2. Miles H. Robinson, *Executive Health,* vol. XI, no. 6.
3. Carlton Fredericks and Herman Goodman, *Low Bood Sugar and You* (New York: Grosset and Dunlap, Inc., 1969), pp. 20, 21.
4. William Cole, *Today's Health,* November 1968.
5. Roberts, *Traffic Accidents,* quoted by Bricklin, *Prevention.*
6. Ibid.
7. Ralph Bolton, "Aggression and Hypoglycemia Among the Qolla," A Study in Psychological Anthropology (Claremont, CA: Department of Anthropology, Pomona College, 1972).

Chapter 23

1. Cheraskin and Ringsdorf, *Psycho-Dietetics,* p. 51.
2. Ibid., pp. 51, 52.
3. Ibid., p. 52.
4. *Arizona Republic,* March 1975.

Chapter 24

1. "Chemicals and the Future Man" (Senate Sub-Committee Hearing), as reported by the Federation of Homemakers, January–March 1975.
2. Marlene Cimon, *Los Angeles Times* Service, 14 February 1975.
3. Nutrition Action Publication—Center for Science in the Public Interest, vol. 1, no. 6, November/December 1974.
4. Ibid.
5. Ibid.
6. *Washington Post* Service, 26 February 1974.
7. Von Hoffman, "Legal Overkill."
8. Ibid.

Chapter 25

1. *Illinois Journal-Standard,* Freeport, Illinois, 7 February 1975.
2. David Zwerdling, "Death for Dinner," *New York Review of Books,* 21 February 1975. (Review of *Nutrition Scoreboard* by Michael Jacobson, *Diet for the Small Planet* by Francis, Moore Lappe, and *Recipes for a Small Planet* by Ellen Buchman Ewald).
3. Enterprise Science Service, January 1975.
4. "U.S. Bakers Could Cut Costs by Making Sugarless Bread," *Los Angeles Times* Service, 23 January 1975.
5. Nutrition Action, November/December 1974.
6. Federation of Homemakers Report, October–December 1974.
7. *Prevention,* October 1972.
8. Linda Franks, *New York Times* Service, 15 February 1975.
9. Zwerdling, "Death for Dinner."
10. Williams, *Against Disease,* p. 226.
11. "Today Show," National Broadcasting Company, 19 June 1974.
12. *Prevention,* March 1975.

Chapter 26

1. Howard Butt, *The Velvet Covered Brick* (New York: Harper and Row Publishers, Inc., 1973), p. 106.
2. Roger Williams, Seminar of International Academy of Preventive Medicine, October 1973.
3. Williams, *Against Disease,* p. 209.
4. Hall, *Food Nought,* pp. IX, X.

Recommended Reading

"There is a need to abolish nutritional illiteracy," says Dr. Roger Williams. "The body of fact is available," we are told by Dr. Emanuel Cheraskin. It needs to be seriously considered and acted upon in the light of one's own conscience and in the light of stewardship. The following publications will be helpful in beginning an investigation of what is happening to our food today and what may be done about it.

Many of these books are available in inexpensive paperback editions.

The Alteration of Food

Braaten, Carl E., and Braaten, LaVonne. *The Living Temple: A Practical Theology of the Body and the Foods of the Earth.* New York: Harper and Row Publishers, Inc., 1976.

Cleave, T. L. *Saccharine Disease: The Master Disease of Our Time.* New Canaan, CT: Keats Publishing, Inc., 1975.

Cross, Jennifer. *Supermarket Trap: The Consumer and the Food Industry.* Bloomington, IN: Indiana University Press, 1970.

Dufty, William. *Sugar Blues.* Radnor, PA: Chilton Book Co., 1975.

Elwood, Catharyn. *Feel Like a Million.* New York: Pocket Books, Inc., 1976.

Feingold, Ben F. *Why Your Child Is Hyperactive.* New York: Random House Inc., 1974.

Hall, Ross H. *Food for Nought: The Decline of Nutrition.* Rev. ed. New York: Harper and Row (Medical Department), 1974.

Hightower, Jim. *Eat Your Heart Out: How Food Profiteers Victimize the Consumer.* New York: Crown Publishers, Inc., 1975.

Hunter, Beatrice T. *Consumer Beware.* New York: Simon and Schuster, Inc., 1971.

―――. *Fact-Book on Additives and Your Health.* New Canaan, CT: Keats Publishing, Inc., 1972.

―――. *The Mirage of Safety.* New York: Charles Scribner's, Sons, 1975.

Jacobson, Michael F. *Don't Bring Home the Bacon.* Washington, DC: Center for Science in the Public Interest.

―――. *Eater's Digest: The Consumers Factbook of Food Additives.* New York: Doubleday and Co., Inc., 1972.

Longgood, William. *The Darkening Land.* New York: Simon and Schuster Inc., 1972.

_____. *The Poisons in Your Food.* New York: Pyramid Publishing, Inc., 1971.

Marine, Gene, and Van Allan, Judith. *Food Pollution: The Violation of Our Inner Ecology.* New York: Holt, Rinehart and Winston, Inc., 1972.

Passwater, Richard. *Supernutrition: The Megavitamin Revolution.* New York: Dial Press, 1975.

Robbins, William. *The American Food Scandal.* New York: William Morrow and Co., Inc., 1974.

Taub, Harald, J. *Keeping Healthy in a Polluted World.* New York: Harper and Row Publishers, Inc., 1974.

Turner, James S. *Chemical Feast: Report on the Food and Drug Administration.* (Ralph Nader Study Group Reports) New York: Grossman Publishers, Inc., 1970.

Verrett, Jacqueline, and Carper, Jean. *Eating May Be Hazardous to Your Health.* New York: Simon and Schuster, Inc., 1974.

Yudkin, John. *Sweet and Dangerous.* New York: Bantam Books, Inc., 1973.

Nutrition for the Layperson

Cheraskin, E., and Ringsdorf, W. M. Jr. *Psycho-Dietetics: Food As the Key to Emotional Health.* New York: Stein and Day, 1974.

Elwood, Catharyn. *Feel Like a Million.* New York: Pocket Books, Inc., 1976.

Fredericks, Carlton. *Eating Right for You.* New York: Grosset and Dunlap, Inc., 1972.

_____. *High Fiber Way to Total Health.* New York: Pocket Books Inc., 1976.

Fredericks, Carlton, and Bailey, Herbert. *Food Facts and Fallacies.* New York: Arc Books, 1968.

Hunter, Beatrice T., ed. *Food and Your Health.* New Canaan, CT: Keats Publishing, Inc., 1974.

_____. *The Natural Foods Primer.* New York: Simon and Schuster, Inc., 1972.

Jacobson, Michael F. *Your Guide to Better Eating.* Washington, DC: Center for Science in the Public Interest.

Lappé, Francis M. *Diet for a Small Planet.* San Francisco, CA: Friends of the Earth, Inc., 1971.

Passwater, Richard. *Supernutrition: The Megavitamin Revolution.* New York: Dial Press, 1975.

Vitamins

Bailey, Herbert. *Vitamin E: Your Key to a Healthy Heart.* New York: Arc Books, 1968.

Elwood, Catharyn. *Feel Like a Million.* New York: Pocket Books, Inc., 1976.

Fredericks, Carlton, and Bailey, Herbert. *Food Facts and Fallacies.* New York: Arc Books, 1968.

Passwater, Richard. *Supernutrition: The Megavitamin Revolution.* New York: Dial Press, 1975.

Pauling, Linus. *Vitamin C and the Common Cold.* New York: Bantam Books, Inc., 1973.

Rosenberg, Harold, and Feldzaman, A. N. *The Doctor's Book of Vitamin Therapy.* New York: G. P. Putnam's Sons, 1974.

Shute, Wilfred E. *Dr. Wilfred E. Shute's Complete, Updated Vitamin E Book.* New Canaan, CT: Keats Publishing, Inc., 1975.

Shute, Wilfred E., and Taub, Harald. *Vitamin E for Ailing and Healthy Hearts.* New York: Pyramid Publishing, Inc., 1972.

Taub, Harald J. *Keeping Healthy in a Polluted World.* New York: Harper and Row Publishers, Inc., 1974.

Organic Gardening

Hunter, Beatrice T. *Gardening Without Poisons.* 2nd ed. New York: Houghton Mifflin Co., 1972.

Ogden, Samuel R. *Step by Step Guide to Organic Gardening.* Emmaus, PA: Rodale Press, Inc., 1971.

Preventive Medicine

Cheraskin, Emanuel. *Psycho-Dietetics: Food As the Key to Emotional Health.* New York: Stein and Day, 1974.

Cheraskin, Emanuel, and Ringsdorf, W. M. Jr. *Diet and Disease.* Emmaus, PA: Rodale Press, 1968.

―――. *New Hope for Incurable Diseases.* New York: Arc Books, 1973.

Cheraskin, Emanuel, et al. *Predictive Medicine: A Study in Strategy.* Mountain View, CA: Pacific Press Publishing Association, 1973.

Hoffer, Abram, and Osmond, Humphrey. *How to Live with Schizophrenia.* Rev. ed. Secaucus, NJ: University Books, Inc., 1974.

Passwater, Richard. *Supernutrition: The Megavitamin Revolution.* New York: Dial Press, 1975.

Pauling, Linus, and Hawkins, David, eds. *Orthomolecular Psychiatry.* San Francisco, CA: W. H. Freeman Co., 1973.

Pfeiffer, Carl C. *Mental and Elemental Nutrients: A Physicians Guide to Health Care.* New Canaan, CT: Keats Publishing Inc., 1975.
Pomeroy, L. R., ed. *New Dynamics of Preventive Medicine.* 2 vols. New York: Stratton Intercontinental Medical Books Corp., 1974.
Rosenberg, Harold, and Feldzaman, A. N. *The Doctor's Book of Vitamin Therapy.* New York: G. P. Putnam's Sons, 1974.
Williams, Roger J. *Alcoholism: The Nutritional Approach.* Austin, TX: University of Texas Press, 1959.
_____. *Biochemical Individuality: The Basis for the Genetotrophic Concept.* Austin, TX: University of Texas Press, 1969.
_____. *Nutrition Against Disease.* New York: Pitman Publishing Corp., 1971.
_____. *The Wonderful World Within You: Your Inner Nutritional Environment.* New York: Bantam Books, Inc., 1976.
_____. *You Are Extraordinary.* New York: Pyramid Publishing, Inc., 1971.

Hypoglycemia

Abrahamson, E. M., and Pezet, A. W. *Body, Mind and Sugar.* New York: Pyramid Publishing, Inc., 1971.
Blaine, Tom R. *Goodbye Allergies.* Secaucus, NJ: Citadel Press, 1968.
Blevin, Margo, and Ginder, Geri. *The Low Blood Sugar Cookbook.* New York: Doubleday and Company, Inc., 1973.
Davis, Francyne. *The Low Blood Sugar Cookbook.* New York: Bantam Books, Inc., 1974.
Dufty, William. *Sugar Blues.* Radnor, PA: Chilton Book Co., 1975.
Fredericks, Carlton, and Goodman, Herman. *Low Blood Sugar and You.* New York: Grosset and Dunlap, Inc., 1969.

Periodicals and Bulletins

Federation of Homemakers
P.O. Box 5571, Arlington, VA
Healthline
P.O. Drawer 24200, Southwest Station, Washington, DC 20024
Nutrition Action
Center for Science in the Public Interest
1779 Church Street NW, Washington, DC 20036
Organic Gardening and Farming Magazine
Rodale Press, 33 East Minor Street, Emmaus, PA 18049
Includes a directory telling where one may secure natural, organic garden improvement products.

236

The Organic Directory
Rodale Press, 33 East Minor Street, Emmaus, PA 18049
National organic buying guide listing food stores, organic
growers and distributors, and giving other information on
choosing organic meats, eggs, vegetables, cereals, and grains.
Prevention Magazine
Rodale Press, 33 East Minor Street, Emmaus, PA 18049

Cookbooks

Albright, Nancy, ed. *The Rodale Cookbook.* Emmaus, PA: Rodale
Press, Inc., 1973.
Anderson, Lynn. *Rainbow Farm Cookbook.* New York: Harper and
Row Publishers, Inc., 1973.
Blevin, Margo, and Ginder, Geri. *The Low Blood Sugar Cookbook.*
New York: Doubleday and Co., Inc., 1973.
Brown, Edith, and Brown, Sam. *Cooking Creatively with Natural
Foods.* New York: Ballantine Books, Inc., 1973.
These authors are owners of Brownie's, the famous 25-year-
old natural foods restaurant in New York City.
Davis, Adelle. *Let's Cook It Right.* Rev. ed. New York: Harcourt
Brace Jovanovich, Inc., 1962.
_____. *Let's Have Healthy Children.* New and exp. ed. New York:
Harcourt Brace Jovanovich, Inc., 1972.
Davis, Francyne. *The Low Blood Sugar Cookbook.* New York: Ban-
tam Books, Inc., 1974.
Ewald, Ellen B. *Recipes for a Small Planet.* New York: Ballantine
Books, Inc., 1973.
Ford, Margie, et. al. *The Deaf Smith Country Cookbook: Natural Foods
from Family Kitchens.* New York: Macmillan Publishing Co.
Inc., 1973.
Goodwin, Mary T., and Pollen, Gerry. *Creative Food Experience for
Children.* Washington, DC: Center for Science in the Public
Interest, 1974.
Hunter, Beatrice T. *Beatrice Trum Hunter's Whole-Grain Baking
Sampler.* New Canaan, CT: Keats Publishing, Inc., 1972.
_____. *Fact-Book on Yogurt, Kefir and Other Milk Cultures.* New
Canaan, CT: Keats Publishing, Inc., 1973.
_____. *Natural Foods Cookbook.* New York: Simon and Schuster,
Inc., 1969.
Kenda, Margaret E., and Williams, Phyliss S. *The Natural Baby
Food Cookbook.* New York: Avon Books, 1973.
Larson, Gena. *Fact-Book on Better Food for Better Babies and Their
Families.* New Canaan, CT: Keats Publishing, Inc., 1972.

Newman, Marcea. *The Sweet Life: Marcea Newman's Natural Food Dessert Cookbook.* New York: Houghton Mifflin Co., 1974.

Nusz, Frieda. *The Natural Foods Blender Cookbook.* New Canaan, CT: Keats Publishing, Inc., 1972.

Spira, Ruth R. *Naturally Chinese: Healthful Cooking from China.* Emmaus, PA: Rodale Press, Inc., 1974.

Subject Index

Name Index